❧ Happy Yoga ❧

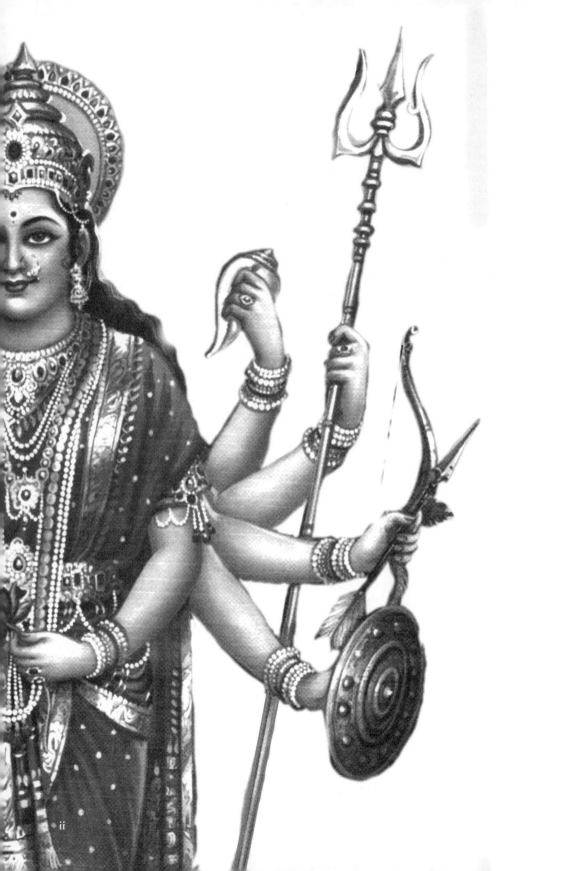

ii

Happy Yoga

7 REASONS
WHY THERE'S NOTHING TO WORRY ABOUT

STEVE ROSS

WITH OLIVIA ROSEWOOD

HARPER

NEW YORK ∙ LONDON ∙ TORONTO ∙ SYDNEY

HARPER

Designed by Susan Carroll

Library of Congress Cataloging-in-Publication Data

Ross, Steve
Happy yoga: 7 reasons why there's nothing to worry about / Steve Ross with Olivia Rosewood—1st ed.
p.   cm.
ISBN 0-06-053339-0
1. Yoga. 2. Yogis.   I. Rosewood, Olivia.   II. Title.
BL1238.52.R6 2003
204'.36—dc22   2003058577

16 BVG/RRD 17 16

 I dedicate this book to the eternal conscious bliss from which all creation arises

Contents

ACKNOWLEDGMENTS

I would like to thank Eckhart Tolle for his spacious clarity, love, and friendship. I would like to thank Olivia Rosewood for her unrelenting dedication to this project and endless hours of hard work in front of a glowing screen. I'd like to thank Bobby Shriver for making this book (and everything else good in the world) possible.

Thanks to Steven Greener and Richard Abate for making this book happen; thanks to Judith Regan for clearly demonstrating courage and profound yogic insight by publishing this book; thanks to Lina Perl for her tireless dedication and clear mind; thanks to Sri Shankarcharya for his yogic wisdom and technical advice.

Thanks to my parents, for raising me in such a positive way and helping me to be happy; thanks to everyone at Maha Yoga—staff, teachers, and students—for your support and high spirits.

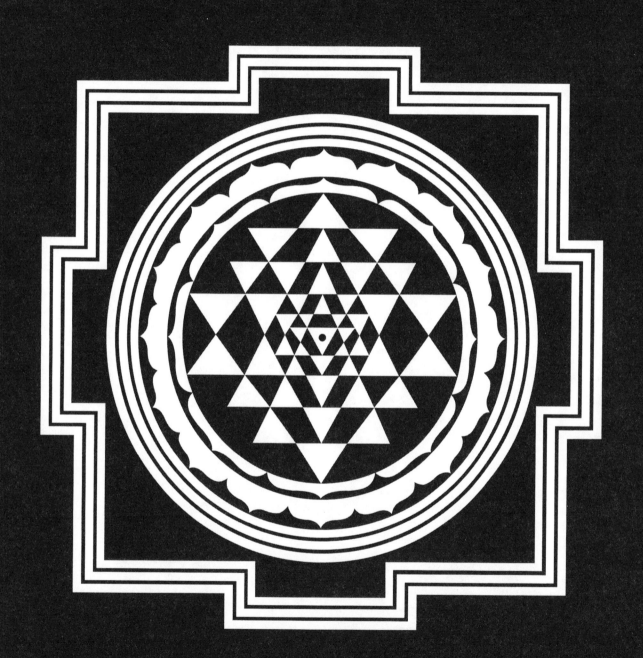

INTRODUCTION

I can't explain how I ended up where I am now other than to say it's pure grace. It seems like whatever life puts in front of you is imbued with choices. You make your choices, and it feels like you're controlling your life to a certain extent—choosing your destiny. But sometimes it doesn't matter which choices you make: Life will keep reminding you of who you really are and what you're here to do. The truth is that I can't imagine a way of life for me other than the yogi way. And whether I chose my destiny or my destiny chose me, I'm grateful beyond measure for the gift that this life is.

The first time I ever practiced yoga, I was eleven years old. My dad taught me to sit in the lotus pause, and I remember liking it very much. My parents were politically conservative, but they had open minds and enough common sense not to knock something until they'd tried it. They were—and still are—into the power of positive thinking. They understood that thoughts, attitudes, and intentions dictate your experience of life. When I was a kid, my mother cured herself of the asthma she'd had since she was a little girl by mentally visualizing her body as perfect. My dad always spoke to me about the power of belief and its influence on experience. Like yogis, they weren't formally religious, but they were intent on getting to the truth about life. My parents taught me to think and to influence my experience through thought. I became intensely aware of the habits of my mind, its reactions, its memories, and its projections of the future. But I was always curious to know what is beyond thought. Through disciplined thought (and its resultant behaviors), one can acquire possessions, wealth, fame, health, anything! But then what? Once you have everything you ever wanted, what's left? After you master thought and the mind, what's next? It turns out that what is beyond the mastery of thought is yoga—the real yoga.

When I was a teenager in Los Angeles, I discovered a few small groups of local yoga practitioners. In those days, yoga was much more of a fringe phenomenon. It wasn't at all like it is now, with thirty million people practicing every day. It was more like thirty hippies in a backyard or a basement. But what they practiced was complete yoga, not just the postures, but philosophy, chanting, meditation, worship of the divine—all of that stuff. The postures practiced now in yoga studios and gyms are only a small, purely physical part of the total yoga practice. Real yoga involves the mind, the spirit, and a devotion to the mystery of existence. As a teenager, I practiced yoga with the small groups I'd found around Los Angeles, and this was how I learned the foundational postures and ideas.

By the time I was eighteen, I was earning my living as a professional guitarist, touring the world with various well-known rock 'n' roll bands. At first, mixing rock 'n' roll and yoga was a strange combination. (I had one foot in the temple and one foot in the bar.) During this period I experimented with many traditional forms of yogic practice, including long periods of fasting, weeks of complete silence, different breathing exercises, intense study of yoga texts, and other forms of deep truth seeking. Simultaneously, if not a few minutes afterward, I was blasting loud electric guitar riffs and shaking my ass on stage in the glorious tradition of rock 'n' roll.

Around this time I was on a world tour that had landed in Australia for a little while, and that's where I saw a flyer about an acclaimed and very powerful Indian yogi. I decided to check him out.

At his gathering, this yogi came over to where I was sitting, tapped my head, and said a few words in Sanskrit. My whole reality shifted. It's impossible to put my experience into words, but suffice it to say it was profound. When I came back to "normal," I knew this guy was the real thing. I wanted to stay around him, learn from him. I knew he had the answers I was seeking. He was going to California next on his world tour, and as it turned out, so was I. I went to see him and spent a lot of time meditating in his presence. Then I traveled around California with him, really taking in his teachings and applying them to my life as much as I could. At one point I realized this was it. Nothing appealed to me in the "normal" circumstance of the Western world, which had turned into a race to get as much stuff (power, possessions, recognition, wealth) as possible, have children, hope that they get a lot of stuff, and then die. The usual "acquisition and consolation" seemed silly. Trying to acquire things, titles, power, status, beauty, or anything else in order to ease my soul's cry for fulfillment ultimately didn't do the trick. By turning inward, I realized I could go directly to the source for genuine fulfillment. Normal life seemed shallow and unfulfilling compared to what I was getting from yoga.

It felt perfectly natural when I said to my teacher, "I want to go to India. I want to be a monk." He replied, "I am India, so you stay with me." Then he said, "Silence is in the heart, not outside. And if you want to be a monk, shave your head." Shaving the head is symbolic of letting go of your past and making a fresh start. But at the time my long hair was also symbolic of being very cool and groovy. I had hair down to my waist and a beard, and because I was living mostly on fruit, I looked a little like Jesus after the forty-day fast. Then my teacher asked me, "How much are you meditating?" I told him, "A couple of hours a day." He said, "That's good, but you need to eat more rich dense food, otherwise the powerful energy will eat you up." Basically, my spiritual teacher told me to shave my head and eat fattening food.

Later I learned that this yogi was known for making people do exactly what they'd least prefer as a way of shaking them loose from their habits and attachments. I was attached to my long hair and I was very into my healthy fruit diet. By asking me to give these things up he was encouraging me to let go of my attachments to my likes and dislikes, thereby not seeking fulfillment in identifications like hair, appearance, and diet.

So I left rock 'n' roll to become a yogic monk. I went back to L.A. and got all the money I'd saved up touring with bands. I abandoned my diet of raw fruit and started eating Indian food and pastries. I joined the Indian yogi on his ongoing tour, and when he saw me, he said, "Very nice. You stay with me now." I played acoustic guitar for his chanting programs and traveled with him for many years. I was up at three in the morning every day meditating, then doing seva (selfless service), then chanting, then doing some yoga postures. This yogi had me study yogic scriptures with the assistance of a scholarly vedantic monk who also traveled with us. I was learning so much Sanskrit—an ancient language—that I effortlessly started dreaming in it. It was never a goal, a life dream, or even a possibility that I knew existed, and yet I found myself training in an authentic and intense yogic tradition for several years, day in and day out. And I truly loved it.

Eventually, the money I'd saved from rock 'n' roll, which had been supporting my habit of traveling as a monk, ran out. I could have stayed at the ashram in India indefinitely for free—I was a monk. But I wanted to be near my teacher, and he was traveling all over the world. As a traveling rock musician, every train, plane, and bus, sandwich, and lemonade was paid for by the tour manager. As a monk, my travel expenses were my own. Spiritual life is cheap, but plane tickets are not. I told my yogi that I was out of money and I couldn't afford to continue traveling with him. I didn't know what to do, because I didn't want to live at the ashram in India without him. He said, "You go back into the world now. Live in the world. Take what you learned here, and remember what's real." So I did.

I went back to touring with rock 'n' roll bands for a few years. The other musicians were drinking, staying up all night, smoking anything and everything, nursing hangovers most of the day, and living the wild life the way that only rock 'n' rollers do. I was waking up at 4:00 A.M. meditating, doing yoga, and eating raw, vegan food. The difference in my lifestyle and the lifestyle of the people I was surrounded with didn't bother me much at first, but after a while I felt like I was swimming upstream. I got tired of breathing in smoke and dealing with cranky, hungover people all day. I knew I had to find a healthier way to make a living.

Then it occurred to me that I could teach yoga. I'd been practicing yoga for a long time, and I enjoyed it. Once I was clear on my intention to teach, it was almost as if the world delivered it to me on a platter.

I worked for a few yoga studios at first, and then I eventually opened my own studio, Maha Yoga in Brentwood, California, where I continue to teach. In class, I play music, we have fun, and the practice is celebrated—a sharp contrast to some classes in which you're not allowed to smile (what's that about?). Yoga isn't rocket science. The only beguiling thing about it is its simplicity. It can and should be celebrated; it doesn't have to be a serious, militant painfest. Real yoga is about transcending the serious and allowing joy into your life, your body, your mind, and hopefully your practice itself. It's about lightening up.

Yoga as it's often practiced in the West seems to have lost this intention. The true aim of yoga is not to produce a perfect butt (even though that might be a byproduct), give you amazing gymnastic ability, nor provide a place to meet cute people in tight clothes whom you might want to date. The aim of yoga is not fanatical attention to the body; the aim is to pierce the mystery of what's beyond the body. In India, yoga is a means to unraveling the very essence of life: enlightenment! I'm not sure how almost everyone in the West has glossed over this important element of yoga practice, but they have. In a typical class, you might get a little lip service to joy, uninterrupted happiness, and bliss, but between the teacher and the students, it's safe to say that next to nobody is actually experiencing yogic elation. It might be lived for a minute, or even for an hour or two on the yoga mat (if you're lucky), but what about the rest of your life? True yoga is meant to be lived. This book is about bringing yoga into your entire life.

Real yoga is not about being serious, miserable, right, or uptight. It's about happiness. This book is an introduction to yoga not just as a concept, but as an experience. It's not just a collection of facts to consume, but a way to shift your awareness of your world. Awareness is the key to everything: The depth of your awareness determines your potential for joy, freedom, and power. Without attention to awareness, what's called yoga is mere gymnastics. I'd like you to get a taste of the real yoga—a practice rarely taught outside of India.

You don't have to become a monk, give away all of your possessions, and move to India to be spiritual or to practice the deepest yoga. A loincloth is not required. You can do it in an office building, in a suit, in jeans, in your living room, at the park, even in a moving automobile. Yoga is not dependent on external trivialities or circumstances at all.

One of the yogis I encountered on a trip to India told me I was a yogi in my last life, and that's what spurred me on in this one. That may or may not be true, but this much I know: All human beings are yogis, whether they know it or not. A yogi seeks the ultimate fulfillment, and I've never met anyone who isn't looking for fulfillment in one way or another. Some people look for it in a bar, a nightclub, a shopping mall, a university, a tattoo, a career, a relationship, a perfect body, or public recognition. Granted, some methods to attain fulfillment are more efficient than others, but we're all searching for it. The only difference between formal yoga practices and real life is that the yogis realize they're searching for truth and fulfillment and take the most effective path to get there. In normal life, we stumble around, guessing, wandering from one shopping mall to another, wondering why ultimate fulfillment seems always just out of reach. The yogic way is more direct.

I'm very happy and lucky to be a yogi. For me, yoga is a way of life. It has given me so much, and brought so much happiness and joy into my life. My teachers and experiences have given me a treasure, and it seems like a travesty to hog it all to myself. This book is my attempt to spread the wealth. Putting it all into words is a challenge; it's articulating wisdom that words can't capture. You can really only experience deep yoga for yourself. And this book gives you the tools to get there.

Ancient yogic teachings say that you are already fully enlightened, omniscient, full of bliss, and in touch with infinite knowledge and wisdom. You're simply not aware of it. You can think of it in terms of radio waves: They may be all around you, but you're not aware of them unless you have a fully functioning radio that can tune in. The practice of yoga fine-tunes your instrument, removing self-imposed limitations. It's all out there, it's only the limitations of the mind that prevent you from being aware of it, and aware of yourself as a limitless being. You can tune into any channel you want. You can have any experience you want.

Basically, you've already got everything you could ever want or need. You are complete. But the mind has created false thoughts that keep you from experiencing this sense of bliss and fulfillment. It's like when you frantically search your house for your glasses, tearing the couch apart, looking through all the drawers, throwing papers around on the desk, accusing your cohabitants of moving them, and working yourself into a state of unbearable anxiety. But then you catch a glimpse of yourself in the mirror and realize the glasses were on your head all along. Why didn't you know you already had what you were searching for? You thought they were lost. You feared they were lost. You believed it, but was it true? This false thought became your reality until you realized the truth: You had them all along!

So it is with enlightenment, that experience of uninterrupted happiness and total fulfillment. Essentially, you're already there. It's just a matter of dissolving the false thoughts that keep you convinced that you're not.

The ancient wisdom of yoga is still as profound and relevant as it was five thousand years ago. The external appearance of the world has changed, but our minds and the human condition have not. Here's the yogi truth: There's nothing to worry about. You are whole, complete, perfect, beautiful, loving, blissful, and you know everything there is to know. If you read this and think it's not true, then you're simply not experiencing the truest, most essential version of yourself.

In this book, I've identified (with the help of ancient yogic wisdom) the seven basic false thoughts that prevent the highest yogic practice: the experience of your truest self. You might think that you're incapable of (1) happiness, (2) true love, or (3) perfect health, and you might think you're (4) not successful enough, (5) pitted against an impossible world, or (6) struggling to escape change. You may understand the highest calling of yoga, but somewhere in your mind think that you're (7) incapable of attaining uninterrupted happiness or enlightenment in your daily life.

When you take a close look at the aforementioned false thoughts, you will come to know them for what they are: fictitious. False thoughts are like unattractive but remarkably realistic masks hiding your true face. Fortunately, they're not hard to let go of. In fact, it feels wonderful. As you remove each of your resistances, fears, and negativities, you will come closer to knowing who you really are. And this is the highest yoga practice.

Transcending mind-made limitations doesn't mean you stop being yourself. On the contrary, you become more yourself than ever before. Clarity, freedom, strength, joy, and connectedness with all that is are effortless by-products of transcending your limitations. Yoga is about revealing happiness, and there's no suffering in that. There's fun, celebration, and joy, and if that's not your cup of tea, you're missing out. The practices in this book are modern versions of the tried-and-true yogi ways. I'm happy to share them with you. What you do with this ancient wisdom seems to be in your hands.

There is no way to happiness—happiness is the way.

—The Buddha

⚛ Reason 1 ⚛

YOU CAN'T GET HAPPY (YOU CAN ONLY BE HAPPY)

In all the time I've taught yoga, the question that I've gotten hit with the most is, "Why are you so happy?" It seems to mystify most people, especially the stressed-out yogis and yoginis of Los Angeles. Midconversation, inevitably a baffled line of questioning pops up, and it usually goes something like this: "What do you have to be so happy about? You're a yoga teacher. I have so much more money and stuff than you do. I have a million-dollar mansion, I have diamond mines and shoe factories. I should be happy, not you." It really bothers some people that I'm happy, a fact that only adds to their already overflowing collection of troubles.

But here's the amazing thing: By the end of the yoga class, the sourest of the sour walk away, having forgotten that they even bothered to worry about my illogical happiness and the injustice of it all. They wave good-bye, with the glimmer of reasonless delight in their own eyes.

In India, there are yogis who have the tiny, skinny bodies every anorexic teenager dreams of. Not because they want to look like gaunt runway models, but because they can't afford to eat more than a handful of rice and a little boiled cauliflower once a day. On a visit to India, I asked one such scrawny yogi, "How are you?" He replied, "I am so happy to see you here on this beautiful day!! How amazing is this existence, my friend, that we are here, where we are!" His eyes glistened, his face beamed. I asked him, "Are you in need of anything?" His kind eyes filled with even more warmth (if that's possible), and he replied through a wide, toothless grin, "Maybe a little food." It hit me then and there: If this person is this radiant and happy in these conditions, what's my problem?

Some of the yogis in India are barefoot, dressed in rags, and exist in "homes" that consist of dirty ground and a gutter. And yet, when you look into their eyes, they're radiating more joy and love than any Wall Street executive or Beverly Hills millionairess has ever known. In this chapter, I'm going to reveal the long kept, well-guarded secrets of everlasting happiness, discovered by the ancient yogis long ago.

Happiness isn't complicated. In fact, it's the opposite of complex: It's the simplest thing in the world.

⊰ YOGI BLISS ⊱

Without looking out your window you can know the way of heaven.
—George Harrison

The average mind will tell you, "When I get what I want, I'm happy." Upon closer examination the truth is: When you stop wanting, then you're happy. How can that be? It just is.

One person who comes to my yoga class, let's call her Claire, was a walking, talking illustration of this principle. When we first met, there was clearly no peace, no rest, for Claire. Even during yoga practice she couldn't relax. Her eyes darted nervously around the room, giving her a distinctive drunken chipmunk look. An ambitious young actress out to make it big in Los Angeles, she knew all about desire. She wanted money, fame, nice clothes, lots of friends, good eye makeup, excellent abs, you know, everything. She was beautiful on the outside, but obviously troubled on the inside—restless bordering on extremely agitated. Nothing was working in her life. Her career track was derailing at every turn; she was single, but searching desperately for true love (she almost developed whiplash from checking out all the guys in the class); and she was always out of money.

Before practice, she'd find me and unleash any number of her life-threatening dilemmas. I remember once she had just come back from the car dealership where she was desperately negotiating for a new green Jaguar. She came to class practically quivering with nervous, excited anticipation. She was hoping her credit check would work out and, if nothing else, that she could at least get a three-year lease on the Jaguar (even though the stress of the huge monthly payments was about to drive her over the edge). Her eyes dilating like a nervous cat, she weighed all the options and considered all of the possible outcomes over and over and over in her mind—and out loud, with me. I asked her, "It seems like you've done all you can toward getting this car. Can you let it go now and be in this moment? Relax, take a deep breath." She took a deep breath in, and on the exhale told me the entire story of why her-credit-might-have-gotten-screwed-up-because-her ex-boyfriend-borrowed-all-this-money-and-didn't-pay-her-back-and-he-never-really-appreciated-her-anyway-but-he-was-really-good-looking. It was a long story. It was a good thing she took such a deep breath. She had a lot to say. This was a typical day for her.

While everyone else in class was quietly breathing in and out, deep in stretch, aware of the peace and quiet of the room, in touch with their bodies' subtle vibrations of life, aware of their quieted, still minds, she'd be doing sit-ups, sometimes obsessing over her toenails. Often she just walked out when the room became quiet.

I'm not the type of teacher to try to force anyone into a mold. You can lead someone to yoga class, but you can't force them to relax. I just let her do what she needed to do and hoped for the best. After a few months of almost daily yoga, she could finish a whole class and meditate for well over a minute. Although it doesn't sound like much from the outside, the shift in this person was dramatic. Why? The yoga brought her into her body and into the moment.

The day that she sat for an entire meditation without doing sit-ups, reading a book, or running out of the room in a frantic rush, I knew something had shifted in her. After the class, I asked her how she was. She told me, "I don't know, I feel kind of strange." "Do you feel . . . happy?" Mystified, she said, "Yeah. But I have no reason to be happy. I feel like I just won a house or something, even though I didn't." I knew exactly how she felt. I explained, "It's okay to just be happy for no reason. There's no need to figure it out. Happiness is natural." She walked away, illuminated; "Wow."

Claire's never-ending list of desires was forgotten, at least for a moment, and later, for more than the moment. Yoga gave her a taste of a different way of operating. Instead of desperately looking for fulfillment in the world, she began to notice it within. When her mind became quiet and her emotions settled down, all she had to do was tune into the subtle vibrations of her very being. And there, within, she found the prize at the end of every quest, the answer to every question, the light at the end of the tunnel. Fulfillment was within her. All she had to do was quiet down to experience it. The things of the world that she used to pursue with so much passion began to lose their power over her. A new outfit that cost more than her rent was no longer worth weeks of anxiety and wanting. She realized she was complete, with or without it. All she had to do was still her mind and tune into her own inherent happiness. Her brief moments of inner peace in yoga class began to seep into the rest of her life.

The funny thing is that as soon as Claire stopped chasing the world, the world began chasing her. She got her desires out of the way and allowed herself a little happiness, but that doesn't mean that her life stopped. On the contrary, when she stopped trying to control and manipulate the world, her life situation shifted dramatically. She landed acting job after acting job, began making more money, and found a boyfriend. Now she's a well-known actress, but by the time success happened, she was already pretty happy in her life and not starved for fame to fulfill her.

According to the ancient yogis, desire—being consumed by endless wanting—is actually what causes unhappiness. Mastery of worldly desire is close to mastery of the universe. What do you think would happen if you disabled the mechanism that triggers your unending string of desires? You guessed it: uninterrupted happiness and a constant experience of joyful wonder.

⊰ FLEETING PLEASURE VS. TRUE HAPPINESS ⊱

Yogis have always known there's a significant difference between pleasure and happiness. Pleasure comes from getting what you want, for example, food, good sex, clothes, etc. But pleasure is short-lived and fickle. It lasts for as long as it lasts—a few good hours at best. And then? It's gone. Pleasure is fleeting, but true happiness is inexhaustible and permanent.

According to the yogis, pleasure and pain are two sides of the same coin. One never goes anywhere without the other, and they alternate. You may eat, but you'll be hungry again. You're lonely, then you're in love, then you're lonely, then you're in love. Then you're lonely and in love at the same time (and hopefully writing country/western songs). Love and hate, war and peace, hot and cold, success and failure, rich and poor, and on and on. But true happiness transcends the pain/pleasure principle.

Everyone has isolated moments of feeling on top of the world: when you buy something you really want, achieve a long-held goal, overcome a monumental challenge, or even fall in love. Yes, it feels phenomenal. In that moment, the mind is quiet, there's a sense of intense satisfaction, and a tiny sliver of happiness is revealed. This sliver is *pleasure*. You might think it comes from buying a new house, getting a big promotion at work, finding true love, or winning a prestigious award. But the truth is that these things just assuage your desire long enough for you to experience your natural state. The happiness is the same happiness every time. The happiness is in you. The fulfillment of desire just gives you a brief glimpse of what you really are. But you don't have to just glimpse. The material world can give you a peek at pleasure, but lasting happiness is found right where you are.

Happiness is in you, it is you, and it's not coming from any external source (including the shopping mall—and did I mention happiness is not at the shopping mall?). This is the essential point: Brief happiness (pleasure) doesn't come from the *object* of satisfaction, it comes from you. This is where many people are erroneous in their perception, and why many people stress out, worry, and suffer: They believe happiness is out there somewhere.

A wise man I met in India put it to me this way: You're living on a mountain of gold and you don't even realize it. Every time it rains, the dirt and muck are washed away and the gold is revealed. And you run out into the rain, scooping up fistfuls of gold and dancing around. But you mistakenly think that the rain is bringing the gold, so you worship the rain, and you make sacrifices with your schedule to please the rain. When there's a drought, you become poor, starve, and bemoan the absence of rain. But the gold is always there, just beneath the surface, and the rain has simply been revealing it. If you'd just dust off the mountain the slightest bit, you'd see it for what it is. Scratch the surface! Look deeper! There's no need to rely on the rain to reveal your happiness.

Let's say you want to buy a cool new car. The advertisements are totally amazing. Your wife wants you to buy the cool new car, your neighbors want you to buy the cool new car, the car company wants you to buy the cool new car, and you know all your friends will say, "Wow, that's a cool car." You get all of this external pressure and consequential internal desire, and you're thinking, *If only I could get it, get it, get it, get it. . . .* That wanting is desire. And let's say you finally get the cool new car! At the moment you get the car, what happens? You feel pleasure. Why?

You feel pleasure because that desire is gone—for the moment. You feel pleasure because when there's no desire, there's no tension, no future, no past, and no unnecessary mind activity. It's a taste of freedom. This spaciousness allows pleasure to dominate your awareness.

Do you think the car gave you that glimpse of happiness? If the car actually gave you happiness, you would always be happy from that car. Is that your experience? Probably not. You may be happy for a week, two weeks, even three weeks if you're lucky. And then it's on to fulfilling your next desire. Your "normal" thought stream creeps back in: *Okay, I've got this car now, but what about the rest of my life? My wife's bugging me about something else. I've had a hard day at the office, my house is too small, I think I've gained five pounds.* Is your car still giving you happiness? No. Pretty soon, you're just indifferent to it. Or even worse, it may break down and be expensive to fix, and then it's just another thing to worry about. Aren't pain and pleasure slippery? You can spend all of your time going back and forth between the two. Pain and pleasure will throw you around, give you bruises, then give you candy, all the while convincing you that each new pleasure will last forever. Like the victim of a nimble pickpocket, you can barely tell you're being robbed of your life.

Now, I'm *not* saying move out of your house, relinquish your possessions, and live in the streets, and that will make you happy. That's not it at all. Living like a monk isn't necessarily going to remove your desires either. *Having* is not the problem at all. It's wonderful to be grateful for what you do have, and it's great to have fun in the world. You can have and enjoy all that you can manage. Suffering does not come from having, it comes from endless *wanting*.

Having is a necessity for survival. Having a roof over your head and food in your belly will not cause pain. When you truly have something, you accept it just as it is. There's no lofty expectation projected onto it. Will winning a trillion dollars make you happy? Well, you will have a trillion dollars. But true happiness? Nope, a trillion dollars is just the trillion dollars. Does having a roof over your head and food in your belly guarantee happiness? No, just food and shelter. You can have food, shelter, and even a trillion dollars, but your experience of these things has very little to do with the things themselves, and it has everything to do with the one who is experiencing them. You can be miserable or happy. That's really up to you. Ownership and "having" don't rule out attaining uninterrupted happiness, but they don't promise to deliver it either.

Remember, true happiness is independent of circumstance. *Pleasure* depends on circumstance. True happiness is prior and senior to the flickering phenomena of the world. True happiness transcends the boundaries of the mind and the limitations of conditioned propriety. True happiness is uninterrupted.

INNER YOGA

1. Make a list of your unfulfilled desires, from the deepest and oldest to the newest and most fleeting. This is essentially a list of things and experiences you don't have. What do you think will change in your moment-to-moment experience if you fulfill each of these desires? Can you skip the middleman and go straight to happiness and fulfillment? Just try it in this moment. Don't make any lasting resolutions. You can still have goals, but let go of the wanting and the expectations. Just in this moment, let go and see what happens.

2. Make a list of desires that you have already fulfilled. Did your happiness from fulfilling each desire last? How do you feel about that desire now? Did the fulfillment of that desire go from elation to indifference? Did you lose what you achieved, or do you

worry about losing what you achieved? Are you still feeling the glee? Are you happier now than before you fulfilled this desire?

3. Can you imagine a life not driven by compulsive wanting? Would you feel more free or less free?

⊰ CRUEL, CRUEL CONCEPTS ⊱

Educating a woman is like handing a knife to a monkey.
—Hindu proverb

·→►◉◄◄·

Everything comes from God except woman.
—Italian proverb

·→►◉◄◄·

Eighteen goddesslike daughters are not equal to one son with a hump.
—Chinese proverb

·→►◉◄◄·

I thank thee, O Lord, that thou hast not created me a heathen . . . a slave . . . or a woman.
—Orthodox Jewish daily morning prayer

·→►◉◄◄·

For thousands of years, in nearly every society, women have been regarded as less than human—at best, pets; at worst, evil incarnate. The concept of women as an evil force, inferior and barely human, was fully accepted and enforced by law. And yet, in our society now, it's clear to everyone (well, almost everyone) and nearly taken for granted that women are equal to men in intellect, the right to vote, the right to personal freedoms, and so on. However, this is a relatively new appropriation of freedom acquired as the result of relinquishing an old—and now ridiculous—concept.

A concept is a mental construct unverifiable in the moment by experience. It is a framework of thoughts and beliefs in the mind as opposed to an actual experience in awareness. Yogis use an analogy of one person describing to another what a mango tastes like: "It's sweet, it's juicy, the fibers stick in your teeth . . ." One can go on delineating the qualities of a mango for days—its color, its shape, which tree it comes from, the climate in which it grows. But this is all conceptual knowledge. It's mind babble that attempts to synthesize an actual experience, in this case, tasting a mango.

Now, if you take a mango, slice it open, and take a bite, the explosion of the senses—the smell, the texture, the flavor—that's real experience! Words can make a feeble attempt to capture the experience and describe it, but nothing matches the truth of being there. That's the reality! Your experience is your experience—the pure, intimate, untainted truth.

There is a good principle which created order, light, and man, and an evil principle which created chaos, darkness, and woman.
—Pythagoras, sixth century B.C.

◦‣◦

Plato, Aristotle, Confucius, and many other great intellects made deeply derogatory remarks—on the record—about women. It's not just the unwashed, uneducated masses that uphold ridiculous, harmful mind-made limitations as truth. We are all susceptible to the lunacy of concepts. The ability to stay true to your personal experience and not fall victim to inane societal conventions has nothing to do with the power of the intellect. A concept will attempt to creep into anyone's psyche, genius or not. The mind of a genius might be even more susceptible because it can find a way to thoroughly justify any point of view. But what the heart knows to be true, what you know deep in your bones, and what you have personally experienced will be closer to the truth than any dry, secondhand delusion. The world is still changing as a result of the recognition and removal of limited and damaging concepts about women. The natural effect of the dissolution of a concept—any concept—is enhanced freedom and happiness.

Concepts are in the mind. They are inferred and often useless and illusory. Experience is the real thing; it occurs in the present moment. Concepts are labels that keep us thinking *about* the world, thereby preventing us from experiencing the world *as it is*. The experience is the God/Universal Energy/Source version of the world: the truth.

Examples of bizarre but widely accepted concepts are voluminous: the conviction that the world is flat, that the universe revolves around the earth (Galileo was sentenced to life in prison for seeing through that one), the Holocaust, slavery, terrorism, and racism. Unexamined concepts drive millions of people to do billions of things to keep themselves, and usually those around them, unhappy.

Don't presume that the support of rigid, false concepts is ancient history. Many are still in full force here and now. If you can't see them, it's likely you've been duped into believing they're true.

In the yoga world, for example, there's a broadly embraced concept that in order to be a spiritual teacher—or spiritual at all—you have to look very serious and speak in a reflective, grave, controlled tone. By simply acting out these characteristics, you can say or do anything (lie, steal, deceive, gossip) and it's justified because you fit into the cookie-cutter concept of what "spiritual" looks and sounds like. A "yogi" I know epitomizes this popular spiritual image. In addition to the requisite grave facial expression and somber tone, he's got the long hair, a full beard, yogi hats from India, the pensive walk, the Nehru jackets, a walking stick imported from Tibet, and several strands of healing crystals draped around his neck. One day a yoga student asked him if a pair of pants she was trying on was a good fit. He said knowingly, deeply, spiritually, "Let's see." He closed his eyes and opened his hands to the sky for what, I must suppose, was spiritual guidance on yoga pants. He opened his eyes, shook his head, and said very solemnly, "No. It's not your color." So she tried on another pair of pants, in awe of the yogic guidance. He went through the same motions, meditating on the well-being of her yoga attire. She waited anxiously for his verdict. "Yes," he said with grim assurance, "those are the ones." Confident that she had received the ultimate yoga truth, she bought the pants.

Why do people let themselves be duped by concepts and by the appearances that go along with their concepts? There's a lot of consolation in thinking that someone else knows better than you. There's a false sense of security in obeying the nodding heads that surround you rather than your own inner knowing.

The shopping woman didn't give a thought to her own opinion of the pants, even though she'd be the one sweating and practicing yoga in them. Did the yogi in question believe himself to be more connected to the universe than she was, or at least more connected to the pants? The essence of yoga practice is learning to connect to the universe *yourself*. A true teacher will not pretend to connect for you. A true teacher will guide you toward experiencing your oneness with all that is. If your handwriting teacher never gave you a pen but instead practiced writing for you, would you ever get anywhere?

I know a public bus driver who has a deeper understanding of spiritual life than most self-proclaimed spiritual teachers. Spirituality is not in what you wear or how you smell. Spiritual understanding is in your perception and experience. Tone and pretense may be in harmony with the concept of how "spiritual" supposedly looks and sounds, but that's just a plastic mango. A nice-looking rendition to be sure, but you have to bite it yourself if you really want to know anything.

One deeply embedded concept is what I like to call the rich people fantasy: "If I could just get more money, then I would be happy." "Just one more credit card, and then I'll be fulfilled." "If I could afford to live like movie stars do, I'd finally have some peace and happiness." "If I can reach my next financial goal, then I'll be at peace." "If I could just afford to purchase everything I'll ever want, I'll finally be somebody." And then there's the famous people fantasy: "If only someone would discover me and make me into a superstar, then I'd be really happy." These concepts are perpetuated by movie star magazines and the fantastic performances given by celebrities in interviews and other public appearances—which could convince anyone that the rich and famous are truly, deeply, perfectly happy people.

If these concepts are reality, then logically the people with the most money, the most fame, are the happiest. Is that so? Michael Jackson? Britney Spears? Mike Tyson? Donald Trump? Often, the reality cannot be escaped, even in the public eye. Pick someone rich and famous and scratch the surface of their image—you'll find that they are often more troubled now than when they were average and anonymous.

Who are the happiest people in the world? Probably three-year-olds. Why? Because they're completely in the moment, without emotional baggage from the past or anxiety about the future—in awe of all that is and above all else, very unafraid.

The effect of entire societies being sucked into concepts, as opposed to trusting their own experience, is extremely dangerous. It's not far from the parable of "The Emperor's New Clothes." The tailor with no fabric sets up the conceit that only those who are very wise can see the "magical thread" of the emperor's new outfit. This "concept" spreads like wildfire—as concepts often do—so that by the time the emperor prances down Main Street buck naked, no one in the entire kingdom dares to trust their own experience. Disregarding what they see with their own eyes and afraid of not belonging to the "wise" congregation, they all participate in a conceptual reality—a lie: "Oh, yes, his new clothes are beautiful." Everyone is having the same experience— seeing the emperor's glaring nakedness—and experiencing the same lack of trust in their perception. Every person is operating on fear. And a crowd operating on fear becomes a mob. What are they so afraid of? They are afraid of not being approved of. They are wanting approval.

In Hitler's Germany, when Jewish people were being removed from their homes, their neighbors had a sense that something was not right. Yet few dared to trust their own inner knowing. Hitler was full of fear-based concepts, and the mob (which was an entire country and then some) bought into them. This is a fairly obvious example of the danger of concepts embraced without question by an entire nation. Less obvious demonstrations of this kind of behavior are still occurring. The World Trade Center was destroyed by a movement that embraces both the concept of an appealing afterlife in the future and the concept of capitalism as an evil that should be destroyed at any cost. This framework of thought and belief is not based on any one individual's personal experience. It is societal brainwashing. So was the Spanish Inquisition and the violence of the Stalin regime, to name just a couple of many others.

It's easy to get sucked into a false concept: All you need is a fear-based desire for external approval. Wanting approval can make anyone susceptible to conceptual brainwashing. And there is only one antidote.

It's the goal of the truth-seeking yogi to continually realize that approval comes from *within*. If you can't approve of yourself, then all is lost. The whole world can be on your side, but if *you're* not on your side, then what's the point? Regardless of what anyone else feels about you, you must summon the courage to stand up and announce, or at the very least know for yourself, that "The emperor is not wearing any clothes. He is naked!" Be true to your own experience.

The bottom line: A concept may seem like a comforting answer to life's mysteries, but it's not. A concept is a mind-made framework of thought and belief not based on personal experience. In other words, it's fiction. And it creates unhappiness. Most of the world's suffering has come about as a result of engaging in false, unexamined concepts. It requires courage and integrity to admit to yourself that you don't know what you don't know. Isn't it more courageous to just embrace the mystery until you experience an answer that resonates as true? Until you try a mango for yourself, how can you know what it's really like?

INNER YOGA

Do some mental housecleaning. Any concepts lurking in there? Remember, a concept is a framework of thoughts and beliefs not based on your own personal experience. Make a list of your concepts about the world (everyone is greedy, so-and-so is a good/bad person, Iceland is a cold, icy place, and so on). Then ask yourself, "Is that my experience? How do I know for sure?" If it is your experience, recognize that this concept may be creating your experience of the world. Do you like it, or do you want to let it go? If you're not absolutely certain, let go of assuming you know something that you don't. Embrace not knowing.

⊰ THE ONLY PRISON IS PERCEPTION ⊱

Break out from this prison of the verbal mind.
—**Sri Nisargadatta Maharaj**

⇢➤◉◐⬳

To a yogi, prison is actually a great place to become completely and totally happy. It's lonely, oppressive, and there's not much to do. Pain can be a powerful inspiration. In fact, pain is the single most powerful motivator of growth for mankind. (However, I highly recommend finding other motivations if possible.) The pain of starvation in the winter was a powerful motivator for ancient cultures to plan ahead. Burning your hand on a flame will forever motivate you to avoid intimacy with things that are on fire. Disease and impending death can push you unflinchingly toward a healthier lifestyle.

Some incarcerated prisoners have discovered intense happiness and a deep sense of spirit in spite of—or perhaps due to—their circumstances. While it was still under British rule, the government of India arrested and imprisoned a journalist who was part of India's independence movement. With good reason, this journalist expected to live out the rest of his days behind bars.

After recovering from the initial shock of being locked up, this keen, skeptical, revolutionary found that to some extent he enjoyed the rare luxury of having unlimited free time on his hands. He began reflecting on his own life and life in general. He asked himself, "What is the meaning of this time I have on earth? Is there something more permanent, and what is it?" He came across books and articles by Indian saints like Swami Shivananda, Swami Vivekananda, Shree Ram Tirtha, Shree Aurobindo, and Bhagwan Shree Ramana Maharshi. As the years passed, imprisonment became more than just free time. He found sacred solitude, and he reveled in sitting quietly and enjoying the simple act of breathing in and breathing out. He found bliss in simply being, and he carried this new peace with him when, to his surprise, he was released from prison after eight years, when India finally achieved independence from England. He became known as His Holiness Swami Chinmayanandaji (1916–93), a much beloved Indian spiritual teacher.

For some, like Swami Chinmayanandaji, when left alone with themselves, inquiring into the nature of reality and the deepest purpose for existence comes quite naturally. It is spontaneous inner yoga. These are the very lucky few. For others, the study and dedicated practice of yoga starts a chain reaction that often leads to the relinquishment of a heavy load of self-imposed miseries. Recently, a number of programs have begun in the United States and abroad that bring yoga practice into prisons. If incarcerated convicts can get happy in prison doing a little yoga—and they can—you can feel free to drop your excuses for hanging on to misery here and now. The following quote is from a woman who had a taste of yoga with Shree Shree Ravi Shankar in a prison facility in the states:

My name is Ava. I can say that my experience has been very good. I enjoy what it does to my body and mind. I see that it relaxes my body and it makes me feel like I don't have any worries. I felt at peace where nothing can bother me in any way. I felt like my body was trembling all over, it felt like the trembling was taking all stress, worries, and sadness away little by little and I can say it was a great feeling. Now that I know how to relax my body and mind I'm gonna keep doing these practices.

In Colorado, at the Boulder County Prison, when a man named Virgil also tried yoga for the first time, he had this to say:

At first I must say I was not going to give into the weird goings-on, I thought it was some type of religion. But I opened my mind up enough to find out it's not. And I'm glad I did. All my life I have been a happy person, nothing gets to me. But for the last few years [since imprisoned] I've lost that happiness. But I feel just from what I have experienced this will help me get it back.

In Coimbatore, India, a spiritual teacher has transformed a local prison into a public yoga center. The main hall is often packed not only with prisoners, but with visitors seeking yoga practice. During the second year of its operation, sixty-seven convicts serving life terms completed a seven-day yoga intensive. At the end of this time, one of the convicts wrote and read this poem:

> *Branded a criminal am I*
> *An outcast among the refuse of society*
> *An ultimate guest of the gallows am I*
> *Heedless to the advice of the innumerable good*
> *Imbibe I did the wisdom of this yogic science*
> *To those I counted my foes before*
> *My smile the only answer now*
> *Forever in me, love in action and being.*

In a way, who's not in prison? If you're not feeling a tremendous sense of love for everything that passes through your experience, and if you're not in constant orgasmic bliss, then you're in the prison of your concepts, which is a mighty prison—much more real than that of concrete and iron bars. There was a Tibetan monk who had been horribly tortured in a Chinese prison for twenty-two years. When he became free, the Dalai Lama asked him, "What were you scared of the most in prison?" He replied, "I was afraid that I might lose my compassion toward the torturers." If you can become free inside, it doesn't matter where your body is.

In most prisons, the worst, most dreaded possible punishment is solitary confinement. Wardens lock you in a small, dim room and no one speaks to you for as long as you're in there. Most people would flip out in solitary confinement. Most people do. There are some people, however, who might find solitary to be a relaxing getaway from the hustle and bustle of normal prison life—much needed alone time with a soothing, dim lighting configuration. What's the deciding difference between these two experiences of the same place? Perception.

I've known people to actually pay for a ten-day confinement in a place that forbids you to talk, make eye contact, read, or write. And don't even think about sex, drinks, or cigarettes (well, you can think about them if you're really in to pain). Watching the breath and body sensations for ten days, ten hours a day, is called Vipassana, which means "insight" in Pali, an ancient Indian language. This quiet practice allows you to explore your own essential nature with the aim of recognizing and eliminating the causes of unhappiness. With nothing to do, no one to talk to, nothing to buy, no one to lust after, and nothing external to bother you, you're left without a world to blame for your many unhappinesses. All you have are your reactions and your mind.

Is Vipassana just masochism in the name of spirituality? Maybe. But more than a million people love to go on Vipassana retreats every year, and the number is growing. What seems to some a solitary confinement prison torture in the name of truth seeking produces in others reports of bliss, healing (physical and emotional), and massive clarity. Its advocates aren't just hippie dippie yoga fanatics either. Movie stars, overachievers of every variety, bureaucrats, and others hungry for a taste of truth and transformation swear by it. Whether alone time with yourself is imposed by a state prison facility or a peaceful yoga retreat in the mountains, if you take a look beyond your desires and your concepts, you might find yourself emerging from a mind-made prison.

In other words, you might want to consider the possibility that the root of your problems don't have quite as much to do with the external world as you might imagine. It's more likely that your reaction and interpretation of any given situation will dictate the nature of your experience. Yes, you can try to change the world, you can move to another town, you can divorce your spouse and find a new one, but your experience of the world cannot change until you become mindful of how you react. Your reactions can turn a federal penitentiary into a Club Med, or your reactions can turn a two-week vacation in the Bahamas into a miserable solitary confinement. Yoga at its best frees us from the prison of our concepts, relentless wanting, habits, and reactions, turning every experience, any circumstance, into bliss.

INNER YOGA

Set a timer for three minutes. See if you can simply be alone with yourself for these three minutes. Attempt to quiet your mind. Pay no attention to the external world just for the moment. Turn your attention on yourself. Notice how you're feeling; notice the thoughts that pass through your awareness. What is your relationship with yourself like? If each of your thoughts were a letter, to whom would they be addressed? Who is receiving this information your mind is constantly slushing around? Thoughts can be like a never ending speech to yourself. But who is aware of these thoughts?

See if you can just be with yourself in peace. When the timer beeps or dings, feel free to resume your normal, busy thought activity . . . if you really want to.

⇥ **RELAX** ⇤

I did not come to my fundamental understanding of the universe through my rational mind.
—**Albert Einstein**

It's well known that Einstein got some of his most brilliant ideas and formulas while unwinding in the bathtub. A little relaxation and increased blood circulation can go a long way toward creative inspiration, clarity, and physical health. Doctors are now recommending stress reduction to patients with ailments ranging from high blood pressure to skin disorders to heart disease and more.

The intimacy with which the mind and body operate is limitless. To think that they are separate is like thinking the ocean doesn't affect the waves. For example, even if you go to extreme (and dangerous) lengths to suppress your anger, you can't get mad without your nostrils flaring, your eyes dilating, and your blood pressure rising. When you're in love, your breathing is smooth, slow, and soft. When you're anxious or unhappy, it's agitated. The breath, mind, and body are intimately intertwined.

Traditional Chinese medicine practitioners, Vedic doctors, yogis, Native American masters, and many other traditional healers acknowledge and utilize the body's inherent energetic pathways. Acupuncturists call them meridians and yogis call them nadis. Remarkably, almost every ancient wisdom of energetic pathways places these streams of life force in the same places in the human body. Nadis are like rivers that flow with energy/chi/qi/life force/prana/or whatever you'd like to name it. A nadi is like an electrical current. This buzzing energy is the detail that differentiates a living body from a lifeless sack of water and chemicals. When you're stressed out or depressed, the nadis contract, constricting the flow of energy, much like your veins contract to constrict the flow of blood. When you're relaxed, happy, and feeling energetic, the nadis are open, allowing energy to flow in abundance. The practice of yoga stimulates and accelerates the opening of nadis—rivers of energy—and magnifies the life force, thereby enhancing its positive effects. The pathways get wider and deeper, so that more and more vital life energy flows through your body. You become more alive! It's rejuvenating, relaxing, deeply healing, and invigorating all at the same time.

The yogis attribute the shriveling up and deterioration of the body as it grows older to the gradual contracting of the nadis. Death and disease occur when the life force can no longer easily flow through the constricted, puckered pathways. Thus the body becomes more and more lifeless. I've met yogis in India who were well into their nineties and even older but who looked about forty. Their youthful glow certainly didn't have to do with their diet: black tea, white sugar, a little rice, and a few vegetables boiled beyond recognition. Their various yoga practices were keeping their nadis open and plenty of life force flowing.

The practice of yoga postures alone is enough to significantly dilate the energetic pathways, which is why after a physical practice you're likely to feel so peaceful, powerful, and alive. Opening all of the body's energy pathways produces a corresponding effect on the nervous system, which in turn calms the mind and the emotions, and the next thing you know, you're feeling joyous, euphoric, and released. Whereas before you may have been feeling like an anxious bundle of neurosis, suddenly you can experience this oceanic peace just from the practice of some yoga postures . . . and that's just the physical aspect of yoga!

If the physical practice is accompanied by a deeper spiritual practice, the flow of energy gains momentum, creating a cycle that keeps swelling until you have more energy than a hummingbird and you're lit up like a lightbulb. Do not doubt that you will positively glow. Of course, returning to a stressful frame of mind will interrupt this cycle and effectively contract the energy pathways instantaneously. You'll go back to your normal, habitual state, whatever that is.

It's by means of your awareness, or where you direct your attention, that you also direct your life force. So if you're primarily aware of your thoughts, worry, or intellect (that's most people), that's where most of your energy will dwell. Accordingly, thought, worry, and intellectual ponderings will be the predominant experience of your life. As you direct your attention into the body, not by thinking about the body, but by becoming *aware* of sensations in your toes, fingertips, stomach, heart, and so on, your life force will flow into these areas. Your experience becomes more sensual and complete. Your mind might seem extremely intelligent, but the mind alone is an incomplete life tool. The body has a deeper wisdom and intuition to offer. Experiencing your entire being benefits your physical health, deepens your sense of well-being, gives you more energy, and stimulates creativity.

It makes no difference what the type of physical yoga you practice is "named." Whether you prefer hatha, ashtanga, Iyengar, power, passive, or Taoist, they're all, more or less, based on the same postures developed by the yogis in India who used yoga practice as a tool to attain enlightenment. Enlightenment, which I'll cover at length in Reason 7, is an experience and to describe it with words conceptualizes it, certainly not doing it justice. Having said that, it's similar to uninterrupted happiness, awareness of the source of all and everything, and conscious oneness with the all and everything. Contrary to popular belief, yoga is *not* gymnastics—at least not in its original and higher forms. The monks who created it were not getting ready for a big audition for Cirque du Soleil. If they were, they would have called it "preparation for big circus auditions routines," and the postures would be named after French-Canadian animals.

Yoga is a spiritual practice, even though the body is involved. It's not about becoming more spiritual in the way you look or the terms you memorize, it's about how you feel at any given moment. It's about your experience. The point is to transcend suffering, not endure more of it. It's not necessary, in my opinion, to develop a hernia in order to have a great yoga practice. The pretty girl next to you may be able to wrap her legs around her head, but that doesn't mean she's happy, nor does it mean she has a better practice than you. You don't know her inner state. I suggest that you set your own pace and go as far as you want to go with your body. Many of the happiest people I know are physically stiff as boards, and some of the really flexible ones—yoga teachers included—are neurotic and unhappy, so don't get stuck in superficial displays. The real practice is deeper than appearances.

Ideally, as you practice the mind slows down and gets quiet. If the posture is painful and you're focused on resisting the pain, or your mind is racing, problem solving, desiring, and your face looks like you just ate a sour lemon, you may be on the wrong track. If your attention does get sucked into the mind or negativity, it's no reflection on you, your spiritual evolution, or the sincerity of your intentions. Beating yourself up over it will only exasperate you further. Take note, and see if you can lighten up. I recommend thinking of something funny fast, taking a deep breath, or at least becoming a witness to your state instead of a hostage.

It's amazing to see how yoga has mutated in the West. Everyone takes it so seriously. And it's the people who take it so seriously and turn it into a dreadful, hard-work nightmare who miss the point of yoga completely! Yoga is about producing joy. And joy doesn't come from misery, joy comes from the relinquishment of misery. In the words of Patanjali, the author of one of the ancient yogic texts, the Yoga Sutras, *"Yogas chitta vritti nirodhah."* (Easy for him to say.) Translated from Sanskrit, it means, "Yoga is the ceasing of the modifications of the mind"—in other words, a still mind. In a moment of such stillness, there's not even a "you" to know that there is happiness. Afterward, the mind says, "Oh, I was happy just then." But when the mind is still, you *are* happiness.

So, relax. It will do more good for you than you can ever imagine. Opening the body's energy pathways, or nadis, through physical yoga practice, inner yoga practice, directing your attention (and life force) into the body, and actually enjoying whichever practice you do will keep the body youthful, the mind peaceful, and you very, very happy.

INNER YOGA

Set your timer for three minutes. Sit comfortably or lay down on your back. Let your breathing be deep and slow. Direct your attention into the body. Become aware of subtle sensations in the toes, feet, calves, knees, thighs, hips, abdomen, shoulders, arms, hands, chest, neck, and head. Move your awareness throughout your entire body. Don't think about it; just notice how these areas feel. Listen with every cell of your being. Notice the vibrating energy, the life, that animates the body. Doesn't it feel good? This is something you can practice all the time, enhancing your connection to the greater happening of life. You'll feel more and more alive!

⊰ THE MAGIC OF LAUGHTER ⊱

Don't think you are carrying the whole world on your shoulders.
Even if you are, make it fun, make it easy, make it play.
—From the chalkboard of Baba Hari Das, a yogi in silence for more than four decades

⊷⊜⊷

There have been numerous studies regarding the amazing power of laughter. Unfortunately, as we become more serious about life, laughter can seem more and more elusive. I knew an Indian yoga teacher who did nothing but crack jokes—one after another—for as long as forty-five minutes at a time. I first heard him give a lecture—if you can call it that—in India. I expected to listen to deep, ancient aphorisms, axioms, or at least some yogi truisms. Instead, he told silly, lighthearted jokes the whole evening. They didn't even seem to have any spiritual hidden messages in them. I looked for meaning, I really did:

A worried man says to his psychiatrist, "I'm in love with my horse." The psychiatrist says, "That's nothing. A lot of people love animals. My wife and I have a dog that we love very much." "Ah, but doctor, it's a physical attraction." The psychiatrist says, "Ohhhh. What kind of horse is it—male or female?" "Female of course!" the man shoots back, offended. "What do you think I am?"

This yogi delivered his jokes with so much glee, he had us laughing our lunch out. Of course, he couldn't stop with just one.

Two psychiatrists are having lunch. One psychiatrist says to the other psychiatrist, "I'm treating a rather interesting case of schizophrenia." The other psychiatrist balks. "What's so interesting about that? Split personality cases are rather common, I would say." "But this case is interesting," the other shrink says. "They both pay!"

There was just no stopping him—I guess yoga gave him endurance.

A young preacher takes $100,000 from the church safe and loses it in the stock market. Then his gorgeous wife leaves him. In despair, he goes down to the river and is about to jump off the bridge when he's stopped by a woman in a black cloak with a wrinkled-up face, no teeth, and stringy, greasy, gray hair. "Don't jump," she says. "I'm a witch, and I'll grant you three wishes if you do something for me!" "I'm beyond help," he replies. "Don't be silly. Alakazam! The money is back in the church safe. Alakazam! Your wife is at home waiting for you. Alakazam! You now have $200,000 in the bank!" "That's w-w-wonderful," the preacher stammers. "What do I have to do for you?" "Spend the night making love to me." The thought of sleeping with the woman is repellent to him, but certainly worth it, so they retire to a nearby motel. The next morning, as the preacher is dressing, the woman asks him, "Say, sonny, how old are you?" "Forty-two. Why?" "Aren't you a little old to believe in witches?"

Okay, I admit his jokes aren't really that funny, but they're just so silly, and he delivered them with so much joy, he got everyone giggling and laughing, and the laughter gained all of this momentum until we were nearly rolling on the floor in hysterics. At the end of his lecture, this yogi paused and said, "Now that is the true yoga. When you are laughing, the mind is silent. Is it not so?"

When you laugh, your whole body responds. Many studies have shown laughter boosts the immune system, stimulates digestion, and oxygenates the blood. Researchers have also reported that laughing reduces stress and anxiety significantly. Do you ever laugh so hard you get dizzy and tingly? If you don't, you're not having enough fun. Rosy cheeks from a good laugh are a testament to enhanced circulation. From just a little giggle, your body is flooded with biochemicals, including neurotransmitters and endorphins, that can elevate mood, alleviate depression, and relieve stress.

So if a yoga teacher, or anyone for that matter, insists you keep a serious, straight army face during yoga practice, they are a detriment to your health. Laugh while you practice! Smile at people! When you just can't bring yourself to smile, I recommend thinking of something funny. Here are a few of my favorite funny thoughts that just might do the trick in such a time of dire need:

I went to a bookstore and asked the saleswoman, "Where's the self-help section?"
She said if she told me, it would defeat the purpose.
—George Carlin

—⊨●⊨—

Never ever under any circumstances take a sleeping pill and a laxative on the same night.
—Dave Barry

—⊨●⊨—

As the light changed from red to green to yellow and back to red again, I sat there thinking about life. Was it nothing more than a bunch of screaming and yelling? Sometimes it seemed that way.
—Jack Handey, *Deeper Thoughts*

—⊨●⊨—

Don't sweat the petty things and don't pet the sweaty things.
—George Carlin

⋆⇒═◉═⇐⋆

During yoga practice, endeavor to enjoy yourself at all times. Without the joy, what's the point?

INNER YOGA

1. Set your timer for two minutes. Now laugh. Not at anything in particular, just go through the physical motions of laughing for a full two minutes. At the end of two minutes, notice how you feel. Notice your body, your energy, and your state of mind.

2. Now, notice something funny about the world or make up a joke. If you are not able to do this, laugh for another full minute, and then try again. It is very important for a yogi to have a sense of humor.

⇥ STILL WANTING? ⇤

It's possible that just from reading this chapter, you have already mastered being happy. If so, congratulations!

Or, if you're not the Dalai Lama, and you notice in yourself a sense of incompletion or unrest, like, "I'm not done, I'm still wanting," believe it or not, you're on the right track. The very fact that you're aware of a sense of that wanting is tremendous. That awareness means you're not possessed by your desire but are awake to it. Be honest about it. Bravely embrace your true experience. It's absolutely essential to be conscious: It's this self-awareness that will naturally take you to the next step, to deeper and longer periods of pure, simple, and perfect uninterrupted happiness.

Remain alert to the movements of desire. Now you know that your feelings of wanting will remain until lasting happiness is your dominant state. And remember, that can't be forced, purchased, married, or divorced. You may feel completely fulfilled when you buy your first skyscraper, give birth to a child, or dig into some Ben & Jerry's, but that happiness is pleasure, and it's fleeting (especially the ice cream). And your need to truly know yourself is great. When you realize and experience the fact that people, places, and things aren't going to give you the lasting fulfillment you need, this realization causes your energy to re-orchestrate itself wonderfully. Life force flows through your nadis. Suddenly there's a space, an invitation from that opening in your awareness. This opening allows for the discovery that you are that which you seek.

When I was a slightly younger man, living as a monk in the Vedic tradition, my teacher told me the following story. It has stayed with me to this day.

One hot afternoon an owl was sitting in a tree. He wasn't doing anything particular. He wasn't even looking around, because as everyone knows, owls can't see in the daylight. They're nocturnal, and especially blind in bright sunlight. A swan flew up and sat there beside him. The swan said, "It sure is hot, Brother Owl. The sun is bright and I'm all hot and sweaty." "What, what, what???" demanded the owl. "What's this sun you're talking about? It gets dark when it gets hot out. As it cools down, then there is brightness. What are you saying? Are you mad?" "How can I explain it to a blind owl?" The swan thought about the owl's blindness carefully. "Look, Brother Owl, I can see it with my own eyes. It's the middle of the day and the sun is shining very brightly!" The owl was very upset by the swan's insistence. He said, "There's a big tree over there where there are *lots* of owls. We'll go ask them about it. A whole tree full of owls can't be wrong."

The owl recounted to his friends the swan's "preposterous" statement about brightness in the daylight. They became very fussy. "Our fathers, and their fathers, and their fathers, in fact the whole of our community, has never seen this so-called sun, so there's no such thing. We've always lived in darkness. You'll destroy our way of life!" One owl got up and cried, "What exists, darkness or light?" "Darkness!" the owls all cried. And they surrounded the swan and drove him away. But how could the swan blame the owls? It was bright, but they were all blind. The swan flew away, realizing he had done all he could when confronted by a majority of blindness and denial.

So now you know the big secret. Even though everyone you know, television, newspapers, magazines, and even some yoga teachers insist that you can't be happy, that you shouldn't be happy, that you should be miserable like everyone else, you don't have to listen to the owls of negativity. Happiness is what you are. And if you can't see it yet, make an effort in that direction and you will. Overcome your blindness! What are your other options?

Yoga is about revealing happiness. Yoga means "union," union with your own inherent radiant happiness. You can only BE that happiness. So be it!

> *What you are looking for is what is looking.*
> —**Saint Francis of Assisi, Christian mystic**

--->=●0==●=◁---

TIPS FOR EXPERIENCING YOUR INHERENT STATE

❈ Make a gratitude list. Build a case for how fortunate you are. List the experiences that you are grateful for, even if it's only the shoes protecting your delicate feet from the harsh sidewalk. If you're not a Zen master and can't absolutely still the mind on cue, this is a helpful alternative. You may find your body relaxing and notice your "I've gotta have it" anxiety dissipate. We have much to be grateful for, so this should be easy to do. The habit of complaining about everything is just that—a "habit" that can be broken. When you see what it costs you—all the fun and joy in your life—it's an easy habit to break.

❈ Breath. Often when the mind gets going a million miles an hour, the breath gets very shallow and irregular. This not only affects your nervous system, but your entire physiology. The breath is like the conductor of the orchestra of your body. What kind of symphony do you prefer to listen to, one composed of shallow, untalented musicians, or musicians with a deep, full understanding of music? If your breathing is shallow and agitated, it alerts the body that there is immediate danger, a harsh environment, or impending death. Deep, full, slow breaths communicate to the body that all is well, peaceful, and harmonious.

The breath carries nourishing oxygen to the cells of the body, bathing and purifying your very smallest components. Many autoimmune disorders (lupus, fibromyalgia, arthritis, cancer) have been improved tremendously simply by changing the depth and pace of the breath.

Take a few deep breaths right now. Or, if you really want to be yogic, breathe while lying down or sitting with the spine straight and your eyes closed. Starting in your lower abdomen, inhale through the nose, expand the stomach, continue to inhale as the breath rises all the way to the upper chest. Hold the breath in for five or ten seconds, then exhale through the nose or mouth. Do this three times, and notice how you feel.

✻ Laugh more. Look for the humor in your daily life. You won't have to look too far! If you have to watch movies or television, make sure you make the vast majority of it comedy. The more you laugh, the healthier and happier you become. Laughter is also one of the greatest meditations. When you laugh, compulsive thought disappears, and you're completely in the present moment.

✻ Get some exercise. If you don't like yoga class, take a walk. If you don't like walking, take a yoga class. If you don't like either, ride a bike. Or just put on some music and dance around the living room for a few minutes. Why not? Exercise keeps the body healthy and prevents it from becoming an excuse for complaining and needless pain. The body is meant to be a vehicle for joy, not suffering. Take care of your body and then forget about it. Don't obsess over body image, but don't let it stagnate either. Your body has the potential to bring you big fun if you let it.

SUPPLEMENTS FOR THE MODERN YOGI

It's the yogi's aim to maintain the body and perfect it to the greatest extent of one's ability. The idea is to take excellent care of the physical body so that it doesn't cause anguish or distract you from your pursuit of joy. Five thousand years ago, the yogis didn't have health food stores with aisles and aisles of herbs and supplements, but they did have medicinal plants, which they had to search the mountains and jungles to find. They carefully prepared and ate them to support the body and continue the quest for perfect bliss.

As the food we eat becomes more processed and further removed from its natural state, it loses much of its nutritive value. And even if you are eating whole, un-processed food, modern living's stressful pace, combined with toxic pollutants in the air, water, and food, take a heavy toll on physical health and make vigilance a must when it comes to caring for your well-being.

If the body is malnourished, chemical imbalances as well as physical ailments can result. We're lucky to have the amazing scientific breakthroughs in the field of dietary supplements readily available. There are lots of brands out there at the moment, so remember that it will always be to your benefit to consume only the highest quality supplements. Don't be cheap when selecting your brands; the highest quality is worth the price.

B-complex is essential in maintaining stable body and brain chemistry. It's also good for your balance. I highly recommend this supplement on a daily basis.

Sam-e is a potent antidepressant with no side effects. While yoga practices them-selves are naturally antidepressant, sometimes an extra boost of feeling at ease is helpful to get moving in the right direction. According to Gabriel Cousens, M.D., au-thor of *Depression Free for Life*, with sam-e, depression has been known to lift within two or three days (as opposed to prescription drugs which take weeks to work). It boosts the mood, is a potent antioxidant, and regenerates liver function as well.

YOGA POSTURES FOR THE MODERN YOGI

If you want to experience your own inherent happiness, I recommend doing lots of yoga. The following poses all invert the body and will give you a taste of euphoria. The blood flows to the brain and gives you a mild mind-stilling rush. Like opening a window in a stuffy room, sometimes just a flash of silence can change your state significantly.

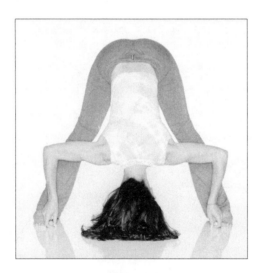

STANDING FORWARD BEND

Keeping your feet parallel, step 2¼ to 3 feet apart. Hang all the way forward from your waist, relax your neck, and breathe. Stay in this position anywhere from 1 to 5 minutes. When you're ready, slowly roll up to a standing position, bending your knees if you want to. The head comes up last.

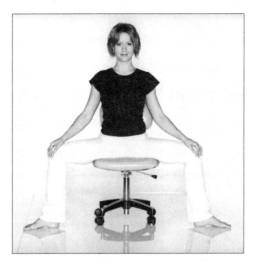

STANDING FORWARD BEND—AT DESK VARIATION

1. If you can, straddle your chair from a seated position, legs bent.

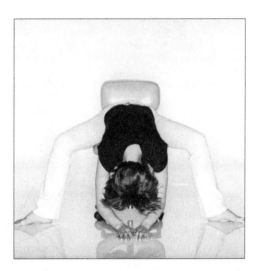

2. Slowly roll your upper body down between your legs and let your arms rest on the floor. Let your breathing be deep.

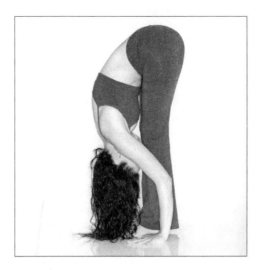

UTTANASANA (STANDING FORWARD BEND, LEGS TOGETHER)

With your feet together or hip distance apart, bend all the way forward, relaxing your neck. Hang all the way down. Let your breath be slow and deep; stay there anywhere from 1 to 5 minutes. If you have back problems, keep your knees slightly bent as you roll up. Let the head come up last.

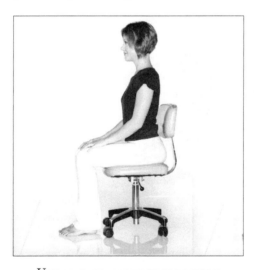

UTTANASANA—AT DESK VARIATION

1. Sit in your chair with your legs together in front of you.

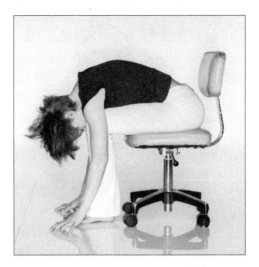

2. Fold your upper body over your legs. Let your back round and relax your arms. Take deep, easy breaths.

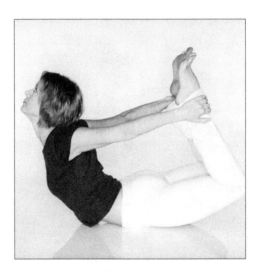

DHANURASANA (BOW)

Back bends are known to be stimulating and invigorating. I don't recommend doing them before going to sleep because they send so much energy through your body. The bow is an especially good back bend because it gives your major internal organs a gentle massage.

Lie flat on your stomach. Bend your knees and grab your ankles from the outside, if you can. Keeping your arms straight, try to straighten your legs, pulling yourself up into the bow posture. Keep your legs apart, or hold them together for more of a challenge. Flex your feet or not—as you prefer. Look up, breathe deep, and if you like, rock back and forth gently.

To come down, relax your back, gently release your legs, and float your upper body and legs down to the floor.

Push back into child's pose by pushing your butt back so that your hips are resting on your heels and your forehead rests on the floor.

PLAYLIST SUGGESTIONS

I find that music and yoga are a great mix. The music that you listen to while you practice yoga is completely up to you. I'd recommend listening to something that you actually enjoy, as opposed to something that you think you should listen to. So take it or leave it, but here are a few songs that I play in my classes:

1. "I'll Take You There" · The Staples
2. "Higher Vibration" · Bob Marley
3. "Don't Dream It's Over" · Crowded House
4. "I'll Follow the Sun" · The Beatles
5. "Love and Happiness" · Al Green
6. "Smile Please" · Stevie Wonder
7. "You Can't Always Get What You Want" · Rolling Stones

Love as a continuous state is as yet very rare—
as rare as conscious human beings.

—Eckhart Tolle, *The Power of Now*

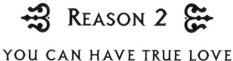 REASON 2

YOU CAN HAVE TRUE LOVE

Have you ever met someone, fallen completely in love, and then after the "honeymoon" period (however long that lasts—two days or five years), you start to notice they're not perfection on earth? And that in fact, some things they do annoy you, some things attract you, some things repulse you, and lots of things push the buttons you'd rather leave well enough unpushed? The initial feeling of ecstatic oneness with another being as a result of falling in love—and I don't mean to sound cynical, because I'm not—does wear off.

So what does that tell you? Most people interpret the wearing off of the "magic" as an indication that their current partner isn't "the one." And then they go into therapy and spend lots of money trying to figure out the endless idiosyncrasies of personality. Or, they start looking for a new partner. And then they repeat the whole experience over and over again with partner after partner, often none the wiser.

But here's the pure yogic truth: The love you experience at any time with any person is not coming from them; *it's coming from inside of you.* It's your experience of your *true self*. In other words, the other person is a stimulus that allows your own love to be uncovered.

It's like eating chocolate. You can crave chocolate, and then satisfy your craving by eating it. You might feel sated for a little while, but what would happen if you just kept on eating it by the bucketful? While you're digging into the third enormous bucket of rich, creamy, sweet chocolate, you probably won't be getting that same initial high you got after the first perfect bite. So was that satisfied feeling coming from the chocolate? No, because if it were, the more chocolate you ate, the more satisfied you'd become. Is that your experience? No, because satisfaction comes from *you.* Eight buckets of chocolate at once doesn't mean eight times the ecstasy. If you keep returning to the chocolate for ecstasy, you'll get diminishing returns until you may actually experience nausea, tooth decay, and eventually diabetes. What happened to the ecstasy? It's not in the chocolate.

⤌ WANTING LOVE VS. LOVING ⤍

There is a vast difference between wanting to be loved and loving. This discrimination is something that very few people are lucky enough to experience. Loving requires no effort. Loving is your natural state. On the other hand, wanting to be loved and looking to have all of your needs met by your partner requires great effort from both people. In fact, it's exhausting—and impossible.

Dealing with desire can be like swimming in a stormy sea. It seems like you're being tossed around, from one want to another, and the storm grows in intensity until you can barely get a breath of air. Each fulfilled desire stimulates five new desires, until you're overtaken by a tsunami of wants. They drown you, consume you, possess you.

Wanting comes from a feeling of lack or unfulfillment. Read that again: Wanting comes from a feeling of lack or unfulfillment. Where does this lack come from? From the *ego*, which is simply a sense of separateness. Because of this *seeming* separateness, feelings of incompleteness, loneliness, and emptiness arise. When the term "ego" is used in our culture, it's generally to describe rock stars who throw things or actors who demand huge sums of money for their work. That's just one expression of ego, but the ego is wily and sneaky, and it comes in all shapes and sizes. To the yogi, the essence of ego is a sense of a separate identity: the me, me as separate from the world and from others. The sentiments "It's me against the world" or worse "It's us against them" are a couple of the most damaging expressions of the ego.

The ego is strangely perseverant. It will even express itself in yoga class. One morning the yoga room was so full, you couldn't even see the hardwood floor because every inch was covered with yoga mats. Even when it's that packed, if someone comes in late, usually grace prevails and a space is created. It's actually fun because you feel a sense of collective oneness when you're that close, a sense that "we're all in this together." Most everyone surrenders to their experience and their space and we have a real good time. One morning, however, Angie put her mat down and walked away to do who knows what. While she was gone, someone moved her mat. Who actually moved her mat may remain a mystery forever. At this point, the unknowable is irrelevant because when Angie returned to "her" place, a woman named Joan was there warming up on her own mat, unaware of any transgressions. The two women began talking, speculating, and accusing each other in unpleasant tones about the particulars of what had occurred. Angie was pissed; Joan proclaimed her innocence. As they stood there arguing, someone else in the class created a space for the wronged Angie. But it had ceased to be that simple several accusations before. The two women had entered the realms of my, me, and mine. Even though the real problem had been resolved—both women had spaces—they kept on vibing each other with ugly ego over the ownership of the space. Truth be told, it didn't belong to either of them. It's just a space to do yoga postures, and technically it's owned by the landlord. So what's the problem? Ego and its never ending need to be right is the problem—every problem.

Ego's not interested in truth or grace but in being right. And in order to be right, someone else has to be wrong. For someone else to be wrong, there must be separateness: me against you.

The yogis say that you are one with all that is—the infinite, the source, all that exists. But somehow a veil has been put over your eyes and you think that you are a limited, separate being. This veil is the biggest obstacle to the experience of love and happiness because it's such a convincing illusion. Like a mirage, it appears to be so, but if you look through it, you see there's no drinking hole, no soda fountain, no shady oasis; it's only sand. Your essence is love, and if you're not experiencing it, you may be blinded by your ego. Yogis use this analogy: Gold can be melted and shaped into rings, bracelets, and charms, but its essence will always remain gold, no matter what its shape. Does a gold bangle think it's only a bangle, and that's it? That would be an inaccurate thought: Its shape may constantly change, but what it is always remains the same. Gold is gold. Do you think you are an individual, and that's it? This sense of confinement to a separate self cannot be relieved by relational, financial, emotional, mental, or physical means. It can only be transcended. Only when you realize your oneness with the infinite does unending happiness become your constant experience. Until then, the nature of a limited, separate existence (egoic) is the cycling of pain and pleasure, gain and loss, rich and poor, love and hate, and on and on.

In the same way, to look for fulfillment in a relationship is to expect the external world to give you something it can't: continued love and happiness. If relationships were the source of happiness, everyone who had one would be happy. Has that been your experience or your observation? A quick glance through the tabloids will tell you that even those people the media holds up as having "made it" (celebrities, for example) aren't necessarily fulfilled or happy in relationships. Relationships don't provide love. Love comes from within you; it is your true, real nature.

Of course, relationships can be a vehicle for the expression of happiness, but don't presume that they *cause* happiness. What happens when you first meet someone and fall in love? You open up. Something about that person stimulates a vulnerability, even a defenselessness in you, and vice versa. Through that opening, fear temporarily leaves you and you feel love and acceptance. That part of romance is very beautiful. But a large part of the excitement you feel when you fall in love is the promise of a happy ending in the form of total fulfillment. We stubbornly subscribe to the myth that our perfect lover is going to complete us, satisfy us in every way, and keep us happy ever after. That's a huge promise! And this expectation is so deeply ingrained in our culture that most people can't see that it just doesn't work. Conditioning can prevent you from realizing how intense your expectations of a relationship really are.

There was a very famous, wise, and fully enlightened yogini in India named Anandamayi Ma. She used to cry at weddings, but not for joy. She could see the newlyweds projecting all of their hopes, desires, and grandiose expectations on to each other, each one blind to the fallacy of the lofty fantasy.

Expecting someone to complete you is not love, it is expecting someone to complete you. Expecting someone to satisfy you and make you happy is not love, it is expecting someone to satisfy you and make you happy. So what is love? Love is accepting. Love is allowing of how another chooses to be. Love is a feeling of bliss and pure joy and acceptance of another being, of the world, and of yourself. Love is a radiant sun, burning for the sake of burning, shining for the sake of shining, asking nothing in return. The reward of being in a loving state is the greatest reward possible: being in a loving state. If you've never been in such a state, then you have never truly loved.

Love does not want, love does not resist what is, love is not restrictive, and love is not judgmental. Love is not controlling, manipulative, or conditional. Love is often the idea chosen to justify these behaviors, but that's certainly a misuse of the word.

So when you desire someone, when you want something, remember that's not love, that's desire and wanting.

INNER YOGA

1. Think of one person whom you consider to be a personal enemy (if you have any). What makes him or her your enemy? Is it possible that the same elements that you believe make you and your enemies separate are keeping you inexorably intertwined?

2. Just in this moment, can you let go of wanting fulfillment from your relationships? Can you allow those in your life to be as they are, and can you accept them exactly as they are? If not, why not?

3. Just for a moment, let go of wanting to be loved and let go of expecting that anyone "should" love you. Bring into your awareness the people in your life and see if you can give them love, expecting nothing in return.

⊰ **LOVING AND BEING LOVE** ⊱

If you've ever been around someone who wants your approval badly and wants your love badly, you may have noticed that the more this person pursues you—or stalks you, as the case may be—the more turned off you become. No matter how much you want to love this person intellectually, you just can't seem to get that loving feeling going. Why? The yogis say that desire itself can prevent one from receiving that which he or she desires. It's only when you let go of wanting that you are free to truly have some fun. The person who walks around in desperation wanting love is often the most shunned. It seems tragic, but the person who wants something from you strikes that chord of parasite, not potential love affair. That "wanting" is unattractive.

And the more you want love, the more you will continue to want love. The more you try to satisfy desire, the stronger the desire becomes. A distinction has to be made between infatuation and love: Love wants nothing except to be loving; infatuation wants approval, returned attention, and fulfillment. Infatuation is possessive and has a sick addictive quality to it.

This is not to say if you're possessive and addictive that you won't find yourself in a relationship. It happens all the time. Two people who desperately want love find each other, and there's a blast of relief because they've both found someone who's going to give them what they want! So for a few days or even weeks, the world is rosy. But who's left to do the loving in a relationship where both people desperately want something? Oooo, then it gets ugly. Both parties may feel cheated because they're not getting what they expected. Instead of receiving love, they're each being begged for it by someone equally needy. From there it slips into dysfunctional normalcy, and where's the fun in that?

How do you become loving? It's simple: Stop wanting. Well, it's simple to say that, but there's a little more to it. It's not something you can think your way into. In fact, the only way to attain a loving state is to quiet the mind a bit.

For example, pets are generally very loving. They're not always ambitious and smart. They're not great at mathematics—very few household pets have devised a method of reaching the moon or worked out an effective way to improve freeway traffic flow—but they do know how to love you. They love unconditionally, without reason. This innate sense of love that pours out of animals is also apparent in flowers. If you've ever really watched a flower, or seen a flower blossom in sped-up photography, you can just see love pouring out of it. It has no demands; it loves existence: It loves the sun, it loves to be nourished, it loves to live, it loves to die. Fortunately, you don't have to be a vegetable to be loving. Unlike a pet or a flower, a human being's challenge is to start from a place of chaos and wanting, and come to know peace. The prize is so sweet, more cherished, and better understood for having gone through so much to attain it.

Be love. It's that simple. If you can, let go of wanting approval. Let go of wanting love. Give yourself some approval, give yourself some love. You may realize that this is enough. If you can let go of resisting who you are, and allow yourself to *be*, exactly as you are, you might feel a tremendous relief. That is loving yourself.

Like finding a muscle you didn't even know you had, once you've found your ability to love consciously, you can begin to exercise it. You can practice loving pets first. It doesn't even have to be your pet, it can be a friend's pet (they're not too demanding). You don't have to say anything or do anything, just pick a pet and allow it to be exactly as it is. Love it, approve of it, celebrate its existence. Amazing things can happen when you are able to see animals with that kind of love. St. Francis, the well-known Christian mystic, would sit in the midst of nature, watching the life all around him, loving and appreciating it. Birds would come and sit on his shoulders. Squirrels would curl up at his feet, unafraid; even the timid deer would come stand next to him, curious. They could feel pure, loving energy coming from him, and they were attracted to it.

You can also practice loving people you don't even know. Sometimes this is easier than practicing on actual friends and lovers, because the intellect and the ego are not as likely to sneak in with desires and hidden agendas. In traffic (if you're not on the phone) pick someone in a nearby car or focus on someone on the bus or train. See this person, accept this person, approve of this person. Know that this person is doing right in their own eyes and allow this person to be exactly as they are. And why not? What are your other choices? Indifference or negativity? What's the point of wasting your time with indifference and negativity? We're all the same, going through the same stuff. Everybody has a point of view with opinions attached to it. Instead of cursing people who don't agree with you, you can bless them with love and compassion as they are.

As you begin consciously loving, you may find that you have more energy, are happier, and people are generally very nice to you. Several modern yogis have reported incidences of strangers giving up parking spaces for them, conflicts in the workplace turning into deep friendships, and individuals who are nasty to everyone else bringing them gifts. Good luck appears out of nowhere. Of course, conscious loving doesn't work if you have an agenda, and this is a common trap to fall into. Once you start loving to get something, you fall back into the same pattern of desperate desire mentioned earlier.

Consciously loving is like developing a superpower or learning to work a magic wand. Once you get the hang of it, it becomes like second nature to you. And people will gravitate to you like bees to honey. Once you've got your mojo going, you'll know it. Love is something everyone wants. When you are consciously emanating love, it not only frees you, but is freeing to everyone you come into contact with.

INNER YOGA

1. Make a list of times in your life when you thought you would be fulfilled by romantic love. What happened?

2. Can you think of a pet, friend, or relative for whom you have felt unconditional love, even if it was just for a moment? What happened?

3. Set a timer for five minutes. During this time, take a break from resisting your world and ask yourself, "Can I allow myself to be exactly as I am, just in this moment?" Allow everything about you to be exactly as it is—idiosyncrasies, regrets, shape, size, everything. Resist nothing. It's only five minutes. This is loving yourself. (Then start setting the timer for twenty-four hours a day!)

4. Take a mental inventory: Are you or have you been trying to get the approval, love, or attention of anyone? If so, can you let go of wanting to find those things in someone else? Can you find them in yourself? Release this person and free yourself.

⊰ FALLING IN LOVE ⊱

Nature truly does work in mysterious ways. The great thing—and the horrible thing—about being in a romantic relationship is this: The love that happens between you and your partner has the power to bring all of your ugly, negative, unconscious programming out of its hiding places and into your relationship experience. At that point, it's like electricity—it can randomly electrocute, or it can light your home and run your space heater.

If you've ever met someone who seems to be the one to give you all the love you've been wanting (some people describe it as falling head over heels in love), then you've truly met your match in more ways than one. This kind of love might render you weak, in a trance—every cell of your body yearns for this person. What you'll find out later is that you've stumbled on the person who will make you the angriest, the bitchiest, the most not yourself. Whether it's a blessing or a curse is completely up to you.

At first, you might notice the arguments you incite with your lover are all very similar. Then you may notice the thoughts that lead up to these arguments are all very similar. The human mind is extremely repetitive. Most thoughts seem new and fresh and apropos to your situation, but really, only the names and places change, most of the thoughts are repeats. When was the last time you had a truly spontaneous, inspired thought? Can you remember? It's impossible for inspiration to find its way in when you have your dingy old mind-CD on repeat. Isn't it getting old? Turn it off!

There's a part of most people (the ego) that doesn't want to let go of old patterns. Like knowing every word to a song—even if it's a horrible, badly written song—you know the words. There's a soothing familiarity to repeating the same relationship and problems over and over and over again. You may find this familiarity comforting, just like the habitually abused find abuse comforting. God forbid you should be released from your mind-made limitations. What would happiness be like? Will you know what to say? What will you wear? This fear of the unknown is a trick of the crafty ego. Don't fall for it. In truth, everything is unknown—including this very moment!

Circus elephants are trained by being chained from one ankle to a very strong spike in the ground. The young elephant pulls and pulls at the chain, trying to free itself. Eventually, the little guy gives up. The trainer gradually decreases the strength of the chain until it's just a very thin rope, and finally the elephant isn't tied to anything.

The presence of a rope around its ankle is enough to make the elephant believe it can't move. The mind is repetitive. The elephant is free to walk away; it just doesn't believe it. You're free to walk away from your patterns, and that will be your experience as soon as you realize it. The sooner you stop repeating the same painful thoughts and resultant relationships over and over again, the better.

If you want to be happy, the best thing you can do is thank, forgive, and consciously love your partner—and everyone else, for that matter—for being themselves (even if they seem absolutely evil). By not blaming them, but accepting them exactly as they are, you will begin to see that what was bothering you about them was really— well, there's no easy way to put this—you. Observe the negativity that might start pouring out of you. Don't cling to your own negativity: let it go. People are going to do what they're programmed to do, especially if they're unconscious, but you can use the stimulation of a tumultuous love affair to wake up. What's in you that led you to this person, to this moment? Let it come up, let it go. I'm not saying if you're in an abusive relationship that you should stick around consciously loving to the detriment of your own well-being. On the contrary, accepting your partner's programming as it is, you can become aware of the programming in yourself and free yourself from it. But as you walk away, look at yourself, remain alert, or else you'll just do it all again. Misery is like a wild dog; the more you run away from it, the more it chases you.

You can blame someone else for your unhappiness until your face turns blue, but the only real relationship you'll ever have is the relationship you're in with you. But even that's not really it, because the word *relationship* implies a duality: a you and an object or world to which it relates. Yet science—and the yogis—tell us there is no such distinction. There's only energy dancing. So get quiet and watch the mind. What's going on in there? Accept it and allow it to change. Watch carefully and be amazed.

More often than not, as you work on strengthening your ability to love consciously, the people in your life will change for the better, without any effort on your part. It's like you start resonating at a different frequency, and suddenly the people in your life start tuning into your channel. And even if they don't, your ability to love remains constant and more and more effortless.

INNER YOGA

1. Think about someone in your life who pushes all of your buttons. What are the qualities in this person that you don't like at all? Make a list.

2. Look over your list. Do you notice any of those qualities in yourself? If you don't, put the list away somewhere and look at it again in a couple of hours—with a magnifying glass, if necessary.

3. Remember your most recent relationship (or the one you're in now). Make a list of all the major issues in your relationship with this person. Make another list of the major issues in your relationship before that one (if you can remember). Notice any similarities? Is history repeating itself? Now burn all of these lists!

4. Anything you'd like to let go of? Repetitious thought patterns, anger, grudges, remorse, blame? When would you like to let go of it? How about now? Stay alert. Who or what is stopping you?

⊰ SOLITUDE ⊱

Settle yourself in solitude, and you will come upon God in yourself.
—**St. Teresa of Avila**

In our culture, the romantic relationship is held up on a ridiculously high pedestal. In almost every song, movie, magazine, and novel, it's epitomized as the ultimate experience of happiness. Although sexual union may in fact be the most intense physical pleasure for most people, if you really look at it, the relationship is not. Unless you both have let go of expecting the other to satisfy your unending stream of desires, more often than not, it will be riddled with drama and conflict. Getting free of this collective cultural conditioning may require some insight and truth seeking.

When you're depending on someone else for approval and love, you are essentially giving your power away; whatever someone can give you they can also take away. There's no independent stability in it. This insecurity leads to jealousy and a host of other emotional problems you are no doubt already familiar with. Time alone, when you're not in a relationship or looking for one, gives you a break so you can step back and take stock of where you are and where you want to go. Take a look inside and remember who you really are. In this way, solitude can enhance your next relationship because you'll be going into it with a clear mind and an open heart.

If you can't be happy when you're by yourself, chances are slim that you will ever be truly happy in a relationship. Taking time to experience your own company can be life altering. Uninhibited by other people's reactions and judgments, you are faced with only yourself and the quality of your own companionship. If you can't get along with yourself, how do you expect anyone else to get along with you? If you consciously love your experience of solitude, it's a relief to be alone. You can find peace with yourself. Once you're able to locate peace and love in yourself, you will have greater ease locating it in other people.

By taking yourself into the quiet, and allowing your awareness to go deeper than the everyday chaos, you are developing a true yoga practice. Love can be a physical sensation felt with every particle of your being. By allowing your heart and mind to open and by remaining conscious as it does, you may experience true love, a love with no opposite.

One of the greatest things about solitude is the quiet. In our culture, as a general rule, most people would rather lie on a bed of nails and then complain to their therapist about it than be quiet and alone for any period of time. What's everyone so afraid of? Quiet time alone is a sacred yogic opportunity. Once you get past your conditioned resistance to it, you'll be able to tune into your own silence, independent of external circumstances. It's free and always available to a degree somewhere. If all else fails, there are earplugs.

First, you are alone with your thoughts, which for most people are constant. You can listen to your thoughts, but they will probably keep going, trying to drag you into their chatter. One way to quiet your thoughts is to watch them, allow them, and let them pass away. Just calmly witness whatever arises in the mind without judgment. Once your thoughts quiet down you may be able to tune into the more subtle realms of your being. For example, how does your body feel? If you look past the physical sensations of bodily aches, itches, and twitches, you will feel more subtle energetic sensations. Do you feel energy in your body? How does the energy feel? Heavy? Light? Dense? Spacious? Tune into this energy and find out how you are and what you are beyond other people's judgments and beyond thoughts and words. Acknowledge everything, allow everything, accept everything. Keep acknowledging sensations and allowing them to change. You may notice your entire being feeling more open and spacious. You're getting closer to being in your natural state.

INNER YOGA

1. Where did your conditioning come from? What does your conditioning tell you a relationship should be? What does your conditioning tell you about being alone?

2. What's your honest *experience* of being in a relationship? What's your honest *experience* of being alone?

3. When you're alone, who do you bring with you in your mind?

4. Quiet your mind. When you're done reading these instructions, close your eyes. Sit quietly and ask yourself, "What is truly lacking in this moment? Is this moment not full and complete as it is? Will the distraction and consolation of a relationship bring me lasting happiness? Has it so far?"

⊰ SOLITUDE WHEN YOU'RE NOT ALONE ⊱

For most people, distractions are the end of any internal deepening. But if you're in a chaotic situation, then there you are. You may be in a romantic relationship that you don't want to walk away from just to experience solitude. Or you may be in a living situation where demands are constantly being placed on you and you haven't one moment alone. You may have children, two jobs, and share a bed with your spouse. Where's the solitude in this scenario?

Internal quiet is the only real solitude anyway, and it's possible to find it in any situation. It is more of a challenge to experience solitude while bound to a dynamic situation like a romantic relationship or a family, but if you're a yogi, intent on transformation, you will rise to the occasion. If you can get quiet in the middle of pell-mell, you can get quiet anywhere.

The big cities in India are not outwardly peaceful places. People seem to be packed in everywhere. Horns are honking *constantly*, beggars follow you and tug at your shirttails, there are markets everywhere, and as you walk down the street, you'll be the recipient of convincing sales pitches from thirty different cart pushers. However, even amidst all this, at a certain point, it gets peaceful. The mind can't keep up with the demands placed upon it, so it quiets down. I've had some of my deepest meditations in city temples that are practically swallowed by loud, cacophonous noise. When you just let the noise be—without resisting it—it ceases to be problematic. Once I sat down in lotus pose on the cool, marble floor of one clangorous temple to meditate. I closed my eyes, and it was as if a wave of silence washed over me. Noise that before was almost bursting my eardrums with volume and clanky clatter seemed barely audible. I tuned into something deeper. It was a great meditation. When I opened my eyes, I was surrounded by little children, talking and laughing, tugging on my clothes and poking at my—very strange to them—white skin. I hadn't even heard them until I brought my attention back to the external world.

The yogis say that any truth seeker can retreat alone to a cave, deep in the jungle where he can't be found, but if he brings his whole family, enemies, and lovers with him *in his mind*, he will never find solitude. The challenge of other people constantly pulling your attention into chaotic situations can be distracting, but you can still allow your focus to remain on deepening yourself. Quiet is truly inside you.

INNER YOGA

1. The next time you feel pulled in five directions at once by your spouse or your children, take a moment—just one moment—to take a deep breath and a flash of silence before, or instead of, reacting.

2. Experiment with quiet when you're with other people. Are you comfortable enough to just *be* with other people, or do you feel that you must constantly be entertaining and

engaged in conversation? Can you share a moment of quiet with your spouse or your children?

⊰ THE OPEN HEART ⊱

Anahata, a Sanskrit word that means "unstruck," is also the name given to the swirling vortex of life force energy located in the area of the heart known as the Anahata chakra, or heart chakra. Through truth seeking and yoga practice, the Anahata chakra eventually opens, allowing life force to flow through it in abundance. When this happens, unconditional love gushes forth, and the lucky yogi with the open heart chakra regains a sense of being unstruck—as though no transgression, violation, heartbreak, or emotional injury had ever happened. If unstruck, you'll still remember your sticky divorce, but the grudge against your ex-spouse will dissolve and be replaced by unconditional love and forgiveness. Politicians who you previously may have loathed to no end for their cruelty and stupidity, you will instead love and pity for their ignorance. The world may not change very much, but *your* world will.

With the opening of the heart chakra, your attraction to situations that will be injurious to you dissolves. Where you may have been strongly drawn to men who disrespect you, women who chide you, or anyone else with negativity to act out, once the heart chakra is open, you gain the insight to avoid these situations intuitively. The deep-seated attraction to situations that end in emotional pain also leaves you. Thus you become unstruck—and unstuck.

When the heart is open, the sense of separateness diminishes considerably. This is not an intellectual concept, but an experience of seeing and knowing others to be not only part of you, but one with you. To look into the eyes of another and recognize yourself is to be filled with effortless compassion, forgiveness, and true love. A state of constant acceptance, the open heart feels like being a mother to every being in existence—you want existence to be happy. Love flows through your being like a powerful electrical current; you want the best for every being and you see the best in every being. I must emphasize again that an open heart is not an idea, a way of thinking, or a projection of the way things should be. It can't be forced. In fact, you don't have to do anything. By relaxing, calming the mind, and opening up, the love does it. The love works through you.

I spent years in the company of a very powerful Indian yogi. A powerful teacher can often accelerate your development, and fortunately, this was the case for me. I did many practices and was single-minded in my desire to find truth. During that time, there were long periods during which I felt completely in love. But it wasn't a love with a form or some narrow focus. I felt in love with everyone and everything. I loved the ground, the trees, the buildings, everything I saw as much as what I didn't see. I was just in a state of unyielding love that didn't need a focus or a person to pull it out of me. Right underneath your thoughts and negative emotions exists an ocean of love. One has but to quiet the mind to experience it.

INNER YOGA

1. Can you let go of wanting to fix the negative people in your life and love them just as they are (even if it's from a distance)?

2. Bring your attention to your heart area. How does it feel? Consciously soften the energy around your heart. Relax. Take a deep breath. Allow whatever comes up for you to be there. Accept it, and let it go.

3. From a quiet, loving place, bless all of creation. Just quiet the mind and send love out to the ends of the universe. There's no need to have a goal in mind, nor is it necessary to have an object for your love. Just send love out unconditionally. Don't worry, you won't run out. What you give is what you get! This is an exercise to strengthen your ability to love. As long as it's unconditional with no ulterior motives, the more you give, the more you'll have to give.

◁ PARTNER YOGA ▷

Man and woman mate because he starts where she leaves off. They each have what the other lacks: They are perfect physical complements to each other. Physical union is pleasurable because a certain polarity, or separateness, is alleviated for a moment. Duality is inherent in all earthly experience: Winter is the perfect complement for summer, hot is the other side of cold. How would you come to appreciate light without the experience of dark? Without sickness, how would you know health, and without limitation, how could you know freedom?

Lots of people dream of one day meeting their soul mate. The truth is that every soul is already mated in the highest, most divine way. Truly finding your soul mate is truly finding yourself. This may not be the way that you're accustomed to considering it, but all of existence is pointing toward this union: the joining of two opposites at the highest level, the finite merging with the infinite. *Yoga,* which is Sanskrit for "union," is the true mating of the soul. This mating is the transcendence of the experience of being only a body, mind, history, future, and person that is born and will someday die. You are still those things, but you also experience yourself as an eternal soul, a spirit free of confinement, one with everything in existence. It's the ultimate, blissful marriage. Your life partner is the divine aspect of you, forever and ever. That's the ultimate completion and mating of the soul. In this state, it's clear that everything is bliss.

How do you mate with the divine aspect of yourself? Yoga. To really attain this kind of wholeness requires unstoppable devotion to truth seeking and enlightenment. Honestly, not everyone has this devotion. Some people will continue to seek fulfillment in a union with a hot new pair of jeans or a whiskey and Coke, not the divine. Those who do have devotional fervor for the ultimate truth sometimes got their initial taste of the divine from a psychedelic experience, the act of giving birth, or even amazing sex. Others who are fully devoted to freedom have become that way from pain or an intense lack of freedom. Enough unhappiness will send anyone on a search for something deeper, something real. To be hungry for the divine with this kind of intensity promises reward. In fact, the yogis say that when your desire for freedom is your one and only remaining desire, you become free.

It isn't necessary to be on this quest alone. On the contrary, a loving and supportive partner can be incredibly helpful, especially if he or she is also seeking to be free of limitations. The sanctuary of a loving relationship provides encouragement and sustenance to stay focused on the truth; it's precious to have that kind of partner, especially in a world of distractions.

Some sensible advice: Every yogi throughout all time has expressed the importance of keeping good company, and this is especially true in romantic relationships. If you're focusing on a deep spiritual journey but your partner's sole interest is the shopping mall, you may be looking at trouble. While it may seem noble to get involved with someone ensnared in confusion and neurosis, being a savior requires more talent than most presume. It's wonderful to help people, but not at your own expense. Getting sucked into chaos isn't that difficult, but pulling yourself out of it is like climbing out of quicksand. Ramakrishna, a famous Indian yogi, often said, "When a tree is little, it needs a fence around it. When it gets big, it gives shade to many." So until your ability to remain centered in love is constant and abiding, stay vigilant about your relationships and living environment as best you can.

Once you've attained a loving state, you probably won't have a problem finding interested potential partners. But don't throw pearls before swine! There's nothing worse than achieving a very open state, only to be bathed in someone else's negativity. Unhappy people seem compelled to squash out happiness and joy whenever it's around them. There are some things you can't share with everyone. One American yogi I know consciously removed the tremendous smile from his face when he went out in the world. Normal people thought he was mentally retarded or about to sell them something when he went out with his natural ear-to-ear grin. The predominantly unhappy often think there's something wrong with very happy, blissed-out people. They think they're crazy and do their best to bring them back to "normal" (worried and confused). So as the yogis say, keep holy company. It really helps.

At a public meditation, I met Cealo, a wise Buddhist yogi from Burma. A young woman posed this question to him: "When I do these practices, I get so happy that I want to share my experiences with my family. But when I've talked about it before, they just negate everything I say and I walk away feeling horrible. My happiness disappears. What should I do?" Cealo told her, "You be happy. Enjoy the happiness you have created for yourself! When they are ready to settle down and be happy too, let them come to you. Maybe they will ask you to help them. In the meantime, love them, but keep your inner state for yourself. If you must share it, share it with other happy people."

INNER YOGA

1. Is there anyone in your life who makes you feel depressed and negative after you're with them a little while? Why do you think that is?

2. Can you afford to buy them a one-way ticket on a train going far, far away? If not, can you love them anyway—from a distance, if necessary?

⊰ REFLECTING TRUE LOVE ⊱

Having established that you don't need an "other" to love, it's also true that there may be one individual who reflects your love and joy back to you more profoundly than anyone else—one whose company you cherish more than anyone else's. If this is the case, enjoy basking in each other's presence fully. But beware of expectations; when the human mind sneaks into true love and tries to make logical sense of it, what is perfect can become shaky.

The usual method of tainting perfection starts when one person builds a case against the other. The mind has the capacity to deaden someone by accumulating "facts" and stories about that person until it tricks you out of your loving state. There are some things you can't make sense out of and fit into a symmetrical, locked-down box. This is especially true of love. Expectation is always disappointed; true yoga, true freedom, is life without expectation.

Love is the one thing that doesn't have a mate or an opposite; it exists perfectly whole in itself. Some have tried to say that hate is the opposite of love, but that isn't exactly true. The renowned psychologist, Carl Jung, took this approach: "The logical opposite of love is hate. However, the psychological opposite of love is the will to power [control]. Where love reigns there is no will to power, and where the will to power is paramount, love is absent." Trying to control each other doesn't work.

I knew a couple who very pleasantly cohabitated for a long time. They both enjoyed hiking, art, fine dining, and listening to jazz. They were exceptionally problem-free for many years. Then, one night, they had an argument because he wanted to have sex and she didn't. She insulted him, he insulted her. She slapped him across the face, and then he slapped her back—something he had never done before. She left him immediately. They both contacted lawyers and divorced. He happened to be a millionaire and she took more than half. They no longer speak except through lawyers at $200 an hour, and only when absolutely necessary. Was that love? It seemed to be at first, but maybe they were just successfully controlling each other and getting what they wanted. On the one occasion when their "wants" weren't compatible, the whole arrangement fell apart. Not only that, but they were able to build such strong cases against each other that they could quickly shut off feeling, deadening each other. By that I mean that when you label someone as being a "jerk" or a "bitch," as they did to each other, you're really turning that person into something that isn't alive to you—dehumanizing a former loved one until they're an object, like a shoe or a rake. You close your heart completely.

Any relationship has a better chance of surviving if you're not in it to get your desires filled, but to simply be loving. True love wants nothing except to love. It's the grace of true love when you can accept your whole self, your inadequacies, your unconsciousness, and those of your partner. You can go through your problems and expose them to acceptance instead of denying their existence. The problems dissolve. Like exposing a snowflake to a furnace, problems don't stand a chance against true love.

It is the yogic way to go through a problem, not away from it. Aim for the center, take a deep breath, and dive in. Nothing is what it seems once you're inside. The deeper you dive, the closer you get to the truth that everything is consciousness, and that everything and everyone is precious and lovable. You develop a kind of heightened vision that allows you to see through the surface appearance of the world. Just underneath the surface, love is everywhere.

⊰ SEX ⊱

Sex can be a pretty big distraction for the aspiring yogi. Like so many things in life, sex can seem to hold the promise of fulfillment. But like anything else, those feelings of intense pleasure only last a couple of minutes.

We're biologically programmed to want sex, of course. Nature has designed endorphins and hormones to be released in the presence of certain stimuli. Studies have shown that typically, men are physically attracted to younger women, specifically smiling younger women. The attraction is primarily sexual, with little thought of the future. If this is you, give yourself a break because it's in your biology. Millions of years of evolution have hard wired you to want to mate with pretty young women, and the media willingly reinforces your biology by brainwashing you with images of perfect breasts, thighs, and bellies.

Studies show women are attracted to wealthy, powerful men of almost any age. What does wealth look like? Women just know. It's in their biology to know. A woman is programmed to act for the future, and she may project visions of a beautiful life and family on a man even before she has sex with him, whether he knows it or not. How can you blame her? A woman's biology is efficiently wired to reproduce and mother babies, so her primal urge is toward security. Of course, there are exceptions and people who act beyond their innate biological urges. But few people demonstrate this ability with great success.

My point in sharing this with you is to encourage you to acknowledge your programming, *yet act beyond it*. Lots of men run around spending their entire lives trying to get rich and have sex with as many young women as they can. There's just one thing wrong with this agenda: These guys think they'll find happiness this way, and instead they just get stressed out and very, very tired. How many women can you juggle? How much money can you make? There's always someone richer than you, and there will always be a babe who seems younger, more exciting, and more pleasing than the woman you're with. It's a perfect setup for repeating the same thoughts over and over again for the rest of your life. To the yogi, that's ultimately really boring.

Women are not above acting on their programming either. It's especially common in Los Angeles, where I live, for a beautiful woman to marry for money, divorce because her husband is unfaithful, then date for more money. Of course, she'll try to get a man who's a hunk, too, but the primary concern is his financial stability. But how much money is enough? How many pairs of shoes do you need to be the queen of the universe?

Even more powerful than the urge to shop is the biological urge to get married and have children. It's very rare to meet a single woman who doesn't believe getting married and having children will make her happy. The urge to reproduce is so primal that most women don't notice how alarmingly tired and stressed out many women with children become! Regardless, marriage and children sit there like a promising mirage in a dry desert. If I had a dime for every time I've heard a woman say, "I just want to settle down and have a family, then I'll be happy," I'd have a lot of dimes. The idea of the future can be so promising. But there is no future. Happiness only occurs in the present moment. This is contrary to women's biological programming. How can you blame a sleepwalker for dreaming? The question you need to ask yourself consciously is what do you really want? Because it's possible to have all of this without the suffering.

A yogi must become conscious of programmed biology and transcend it. Notice what it is you think will bring you never-ending happiness, then go one step further in your query. Has anyone else achieved never-ending happiness this way? Has anyone reached a state of *lasting* fulfillment through shopping, having children, marrying well, or having sex with everybody?

⊰ BEYOND BIOLOGY ⊱

Yoga class is a great practice for moving beyond the promise of fulfillment through the body, and I'm not even talking about meditation and postures. All the beauty queens and high school drama club stars from all over the world come to Los Angeles for fame and fortune, and inevitably, many end up in my yoga class. To the average man, the sight of beautiful bodies sweating through their yoga tights is a vision of unending possibilities. But come to yoga class often enough, and the bodies lose their mystique. If it's a particularly packed class, in Chattaranga pose, for example, you might be close enough to someone's feet to smell them. That can be sufficient to shatter your dream right there, trust me. The body loses its mystique as a desire fulfiller and sex object when you really look at it. Bodies begin to look like what they are—just bodies. Yes, it's the container for the soul, but a cosmetically beautiful body does not equate to a developed spirit. As you learn to look past the surface, you may develop the ability to see into the heart—a much more rewarding vision.

It's the practice of the yogi not to run away from delusions, but to face them. Becoming aware of delusions dissolves them. Take note: This doesn't mean denying your sexual impulses and stuffing them away somewhere to fester and grow like mold. Nor does it mean you should empower your delusions by acting them out; fulfilling your desires over and over again won't squash them. The yogis say trying to get rid of desires by acting on them is like trying to stop a fire by throwing gasoline on it. With acting out desires and suppression out of the picture, what's left? Any teacher worth his salt will advise you to face your desires, stare them down with fierce examination, be aware of them in an alert, conscious state, and thereby dissolve them.

The next time your loins are pining for that sexy redhead, ask yourself, "Do I think this is going to fulfill me?" If you do have meaningless sex, ask yourself afterward, "Did this satisfy me like I thought it would? Was it really worth it?" Undoubtedly, you'll be pining for someone else in a matter of days, if not minutes. That's a lot of energy to spend without much true gratification beyond the momentary orgasm. Just become aware that you're acting on your programming. That awareness alone is enough to begin to free you.

Likewise, if you believe that everything would be perfect if only you were to get married and have children, go through that desire mentally. Ask yourself, "Do I think this is going to fulfill me?" Imagine that you are married, and go beyond the wedding ceremony and the vows. Then what? Then it's life as usual, but you're legally married. Things don't change that much. If anything, now you have your spouse's problems to deal with as well as your own. If you had an expectation of overwhelming marital happiness and it isn't met, you'll also have a major letdown to deal with.

Having children is a beautiful, magical, normal thing to do. But many people believe it's the beginning of paradise on earth and they expect their new child to complete them. It's not a fair expectation, and it usually leads to disillusionment. Raising children involves an enormous amount of work; a parent is a chauffeur, a psychiatrist, a personal secretary, a cook, a maid, and more. Parenting can be, and very often appears to be, exhausting. And in the end, your children grow up and become their own people. Even if being a parent is extremely fulfilling, to a certain extent it does end, and then what are you? You're back to yourself again.

There's absolutely nothing wrong with getting married and having children. If you are truly happy to begin with, you will be more likely to extend this happiness into every situation. Problems arise when you expect your spouse or children to satisfy your desires, to fulfill you, and to make you happy. When you look at anything in life as a desire quencher, you deaden it. It becomes an object of desire. You stop the movement of spontaneous life flowing when you force your will. Wanting to get something out of marriage or children or sex will only take you further away from fulfillment.

The actual physical union of a man and a woman is a beautiful metaphor for union with the divine because in that moment, the physical boundaries defining your everyday awareness dissolve. It's not uncommon to experience yourself and your partner as one ecstatic being, unified, without the sense of separation. This relinquishment of your identity as a single, lonely individual is very spiritual. But it's just a fleeting taste of your natural state. Some yogis walk around in a constant, never-ending orgasm. Of course, you adapt to this being your predominant state. You become functionally orgasmic.

Yogis generally don't think about sex much. They view sex as silly: All the energy used to think about sex, pursue sex, or constantly have sex can be used to fuel the pursuit of the divine. One yogi I studied with was asked, "Why are you celibate? Why don't you have sex?" His answer was insightful: "I don't have sex for the same reason you do have sex. It feels good! Sexual energy turns into love for a meditating yogi." Have sex or don't have sex, but don't worry about it. Some yogis pursue the experience of the divine while they have sex. Isn't that efficient?

⋈ TANTRA ⋈

Traditionally, yogis have approached sex in different ways. Some yogis just don't do it. The urge goes away, and they sit alone in bliss on a comfortable rock near a river. But there is a part of the yogi tradition that advises the use of sex as a powerful tool for communing with the infinite.

You can turn the body into an instrument for experiencing the bliss of the universe while having sex. In order to let this happen, it's essential to go into sexual activity without ulterior motives, expectations, or negativity. Beyond being lovers, you and your partner must be on the same team, friends, and focused on a common yearning for spiritual freedom.

The word *tantra* is Sanskrit. *Tan* means "to stretch, spread, or expand," and *tra* means "tool or instrument." Tantra is a tool for expansion. Having tantric sex—the yogic act of intimate physical communion—is actually a deep spiritual practice.

The practice of tantric sex is ancient and shows up in several forms in Hinduism, Buddhism, Tibetan mysticism, and even Chinese Taoism. But the essence of the practice always remains this: Use sex not as an escape, but as an instrument for experiencing oneness not only with your partner, but with all that is, the universe, the divine, the higher power.

Tantra is not the Kama Sutra. The Kama Sutra is an ancient Hindu guide to love-making (literally translated, it means "Lessons of Love") illustrating postures and techniques to enhance pleasure and orgasms. Tantric sex goes beyond pleasure and orgasm by using sexual energy as a fuel for expanding consciousness. A by-product of this practice—although not the ultimate goal—is an enhanced ability to give, receive, and enjoy love and ecstatic pleasure.

Because the act of sex—physical counterparts in physical union—is a natural metaphor for form communing with the infinite formless, it can be a yogic practice for deepening the awareness of oneness with all that is. During tantric sex, the idea is that the lovers realize the perfect union of opposites in themselves.

The techniques prescribed for practicing tantric sex are as varied as the people who discovered them: The Tibetans, Jains, Hindus, Buddhists, Taoists, and southern California New Agers all have their own very detailed instruction manuals for where to put what, for how long, what to say to each other, what color sheets to put on the bed, and what to eat before, during, and after. This is all good and well, but the purpose of this practice is your *experience*, not your adherence to a do-it-yourself, dress-and-eat-to-impress-for-enlightenment guidebook. So I'll share the basics with you and leave the rest up to you.

First, become aware that the root of tantra is the interconnectedness of all existence. The core of tantra revolves around the eternal truth that as above, so below, as within, so without—the microcosm is a true representation of the bigger picture. Yogis say that if even a drop of water is missing, all of creation will thirst. If you inflict negativity on a papaya tree, you have harmed millions of stars. Your life is not a mechanical, separate entity, it is part of a vast, whole existence that is not only connected but one. This truth applies on every level: to the physical body, the emotional body, and the spiritual body. There is no spot where this truth is not. Everything is deeply related to everything else. *You* are deeply related to everything else.

Tantra is not the only way, but it is one way. And if you're going to be having sex anyway, why not investigate the deeper dimensions of this dance rather than remaining in the shallow water with everybody else?

RIDING THE WAVE

Among Americans, the average time spent lovemaking is reportedly 28.1 minutes. In tantric sex, that time is extended for as long as twelve hours. There are legends of extending it for days, but don't try this right off the bat. The basic tantric method is very simple: Become intensely present in the ecstatic moment just before the orgasmic climax. There's a lot of energy pushing your being toward pleasure gratification at that time, and that's the energy that's redirected toward union with the infinite. There's nothing for you to do except remain open. In fact, it's more of a not doing than anything else. Your *intention* to experience the divine, as opposed to immediate gratification, is enough to allow deep waves of bliss to pass through your awareness, bringing a sense of oneness with the entire universe, not to mention your partner.

Take your time reaching the tantra zone. In tantric sex, there's no hurry. As with all yogic practices, tantra is not a serious, melancholy, heavyhearted ordeal. It's joy and celebration in the pursuit of deeper bliss. So don't get uptight about it. Enjoy each other!

When practicing tantra, there's an advantage to staying with the same partner for long periods of time: Your energies naturally harmonize. Not only do you experience lovemaking as one very happy being, you experience a union with the absolute as well. You become aware of yourself as a united partnership, and you become aware of yourself as form united with the formless. After a while, the bliss that you experience during tantric sex will be so much more intense than an orgasm that you may find yourself sated by it. In other words, after a few hours of lovemaking, whether you reach orgasm or not becomes irrelevant. You hover, float, drift, sail; you're melting ice, you're the entire ocean. Boundaries dissolve, beingness opens. There's no more fight, there's no one left to fight, you are everyone, and everyone's you, immersed in glowing, blessing waters of effortless forgiveness and acceptance.

Tantra is essentially a practice of spiritualizing sexuality, enhancing and heightening your awareness of yourself. I've shared the basics with you. Observe your own experience. Do with it what you will.

The truth of the Universe can only be realized within the framework of the human body.
—The Buddha

⊷►◉◄⊶

TIPS FOR EXPERIENCING TRUE LOVE

❋ Loving requires no effort. Desperately wanting love is exhausting. Why not do yourself a favor and let the world off the hook? *Be* the love you want, *be* the approval you want. Try loving the world and see how much easier your life gets.

❋ The ego needs enemies. Me or us against them—and all other separateness—is a trick of the ego. We're all in this together. Truth, grace, and forgiveness facilitate healing on every level.

❋ Wanting is repellent. When you realize you are love, love will fly to you from every direction. As long as you are in a lacking mind-set, you are a lack magnet.

❋ Practice loving. Anybody, even people you don't know, can be a target for your loving energy. Start exercising your power to love unconditionally. Take the emphasis off of getting love and put it on giving love.

❋ Expectation will always be disappointed. Why not let the people in your life, especially your life partner, be as they are? They have to go through whatever their life demands of them. Can you love them without wanting them to be anything other than what they are? Can you love them without controlling them?

❋ Observe your unconscious behavior. Stay alert. Are you a slave to your biological programming? Are you sure that's working for you?

❋ Always love and support your partner. Your partner is you and you are your partner, so be helpful, be loving.

SUPPLEMENTS FOR LOVE

L-Phenylalanine stimulates the nervous system, elevates mood, and assists cognition. This supplement plays an important role in memory and alertness and has a similar effect on the emotional experience as chocolate. You can increase its effectiveness by also taking vitamin B-complex (50–100mg/day). L-phenylalanine is readily available in any good health food store.

Yohimbe is a natural, herbal aphrodisiac. It increases circulation in the pelvic region and enhances sexual response in both men and women.

POSTURES FOR THE HEART CHAKRA

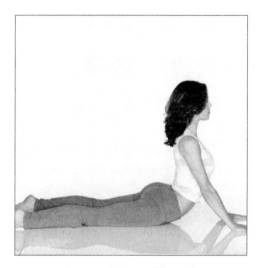

BHUJANGASANA (COBRA)

Lie flat on your stomach. Bring your hands, palms down, next to your shoulders (more or less, depending on your flexibility). Keeping them flat, push down with your palms, raising your upper body. Keep your elbows close to your body, shoulders down and back, chest forward. Push your pubic bone down, the tops of your feet down, legs straight, knees stay on the floor. Breathe in deeply through your nose. Look up unless it hurts your neck, in which case don't worry about it. Keep your palms flat and hold this position for 30 seconds to a minute. Slowly come down, turning your head to one side, and relax. Repeat 3 times.

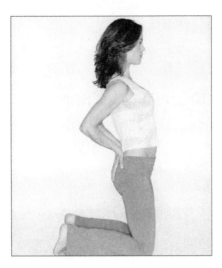

USTRASANA (CAMEL)

1. From a kneeling position, push your hips forward, lift your chest and put your hands either on your lower back, hips, waist, or the top of your butt.

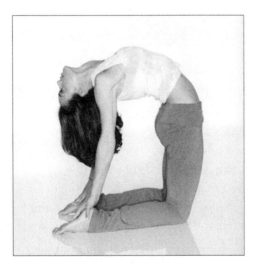

2. Arch back as far as you can and bring your hands to your heels or the soles of your feet. If you can't reach your heels, tuck your toes under, elevating your heels, and see if you can reach them this way. If you can't, don't worry about it; just go back as far as you can. Hold this position for a minute, taking full, deep breaths. *Slowly* come back up the way you went down. Then fold forward into child's pose.

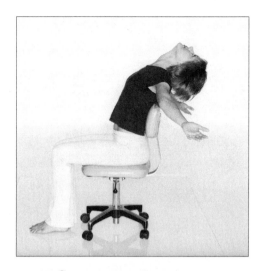

CAMEL—AT DESK VARIATION

Sitting in a normal office chair, open your arms wide and arch your upper back just over the top of the desk chair, keeping the rest of your back upright and supported by your stomach. Let your head fall back between your shoulder blades and take full easy breaths.

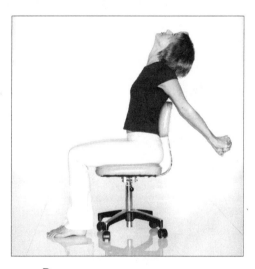

BACKBEND—AT DESK VARIATION

Sitting in your chair, clasp your hands behind your back and straighten your arms. Drop your head back and lift your chest.

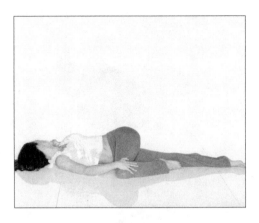

TWIST

It's a good idea to do a gentle twist after these postures. Lie flat on your back. Pull your left knee to your chest and squeeze it in. Slowly drop your bent left leg over your straight right leg. Look over your left shoulder, push your right shoulder down, and keep the ball of your left foot roughly around your right kneecap area. Hold that for a few deep breaths, stretching your back and spine, and then do the other side.

YOGA FOR PARTNERS

RECLINING FORWARD FOLD

This posture requires two people who cooperate well (this is very important).

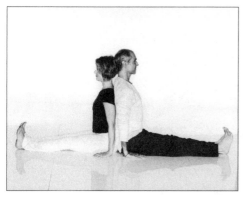

1. Sit back to back, legs straight in front.

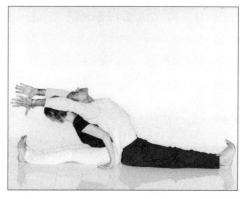

2. Keep your feet flexed as partner number 1 folds forward into a sitting forward bend. Partner number 2 leans back, reclining on number 1.

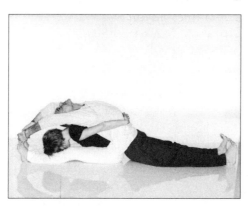

3. Partner number 2 can reach his or her arms up and behind their head, clasping number 1's big toes with the thumb and forefinger. If number 1 is very flexible, he or she can reach his or her arms behind, gently pulling number 2 around the waist and pulling him or her into a deeper back bend.

This posture is a gentle back bend for number 2 that opens the heart area and shoulders. For number 1, it's a chance to go deeper into a forward bend with the weight of number 2's body. Stay in the pose for 2 or 3 minutes and notice how the pose deepens as your breath deepens. You can also try synchronizing your breathing and tuning into your partner's energy. To switch roles, slowly come out of it; then number 1 leans back as number 2 goes into the forward bend.

PLAYLIST SUGGESTIONS

1. "No More Drama" · Mary J. Blige
2. "Best of My Love" · The Emotions
3. "Sumthin' Sumthin'" · Maxwell
4. "Don't Worry, Baby" · The Beach Boys
5. "Ring of Fire" · Johnny Cash
6. "Sexual Healing" · Marvin Gaye
7. "Let's Stay Together" · Al Green
8. "Use Me" · Bill Withers
9. "My Romance" · James Taylor
10. "Say a Little Prayer" · Aretha Franklin
11. "Crazy Love" · Van Morrison

To identify oneself with the body and yet seek happiness
is like attempting to cross a river on the back of an alligator.
In truth, you are spirit.

—Ramana Maharshi

✷ REASON 3 ✷

YOU'RE NOT FAT (AND NEITHER AM I)

There is one question that seems to be at the heart of every yogic practice, and it is "What are you?" For many yogis, it seems that what you truly believe yourself to be dictates how you experience yourself. So, if you think that what you are is fat or a fat person, that will be your primary experience of yourself. Believing it and thinking it reinforces your condition. But is that really what you are? When you tap into your essence and find out what you really are, it frees you from being locked into this kind of limited experience (thinking or experiencing yourself to be fat). Once you know what you truly are, changing the size and shape of your body will be as easy as taking off a red hat and putting on a blue one.

Consider the possibility that you're not what you think you are. It's true that you might seem to be a person, but what is a person? You may seem to be a body, but what is a body? And you may seem to be flesh and blood, but that's just a point of view, because what is flesh and blood?

In a basic science class, we learn that all matter—everything—is composed of different combinations of elements. This fact applies to the human body as well. What are you? Approximately 65 percent oxygen (roughly 97 pounds of a 150-pound body), 3 percent nitrogen (5 pounds), 0.25 percent sulfur (3 ¼ ounces), 10 percent hydrogen (15 pounds), and so on. The body is made only of these elements in different combinations. Your hair, your eyes, your various fluids, your skin, your feet, your intestines—and even your fat—are made up of elements. If you poured all of the elements that make up a human body into a sack, never in a million years would you get a person. You'd just get a sack of chemicals. And yet technically that's what we seem to be: a sack of chemicals.

Also in a basic science class, it's made clear that these elements are made entirely of atoms—electrons, neutrons, and protons. That's it. The way that these elements are distinguished from one another depends on the pattern in which the atoms are arranged. Everything in the universe is composed of electrons, neutrons, and protons, and only electrons, neutrons, and protons, including your body.

And what are electrons, neutrons, and protons? When examined under an electron microscope, scientists attest to the fact that they are 99.9 percent empty space. The other less than 0.1 percent is not really anything more than a little evidence of movement, called energy.

So if emptiness and energy are what make electrons, neutrons, and protons, and electrons, protons, and neutrons are what make atoms, and atoms are what make elements, and elements make up your body, that means your body is made up of 99.9 percent empty space and less than 0.1 percent moving vibration.

You might think you are a person with a body and its characteristics—arms, belly, nose, ears, feet, hips, moles, and so on. But what are you really? You are empty space and a little vibration, and that's a fact. For thousands of years, yogis have known that the physical body is not what you are. The body is just a physical appearance; in essence you are much more than that. Only in relatively recent years has science corroborated ancient yogic wisdom with solid, proven evidence. Could you be just awareness, and a smorgasbord of thoughts, vibrations, and fantasies, masquerading as solid matter? This is not existential, because the existentialists would argue that nothing exists. Yogis say everything exists, and nothing is separate, and everything is spirit.

One of the most empowering things you can know is this: I am. It's really all you can know for sure. Everything else is just a belief; everything else is conceptualization; everything else is your reaction to fear. So when it comes down to it, all anybody knows, *really knows*, is that they exist. You are. You exist.

INNER YOGA

Set a timer for three minutes. Ask yourself, "What am I?" Don't think about it. Let your mind be quiet and listen for the answer. Repeat the question as often as you want: "What am I?"

⊰ WHAT'S YOUR EXPERIENCE? ⊱

If you're mostly emptiness and a little bit of vibrating energy, then what's the problem? Why does the body feel like solid matter? And why do people get sick? And why does everyone worry all the time? And why does the body look like a body? Why doesn't everything look like emptiness if that's what it is?

Imagine that you're lost in a thick forest. The denseness of trees and bushes makes it impossible to navigate—you are faced with a never-ending foliage assault. Many people, if lost in such overwhelming shrubbery, would become upset, scream, stress out, and possibly injure themselves wandering in circles of frustration. Others might just give up and lie down to die. But if you could change your point of view, if you could climb the tallest tree and see from the top that you are only a few steps from a clear path leading you into an open field, your experience could change radically. Suddenly, instead of a life-threatening tragedy, you are on a pleasant stroll. Calmed, you may notice the beautiful greens of the trees, hear birds chirping for the first time, smell the intoxicating perfume of the flowers. What was tragic becomes enchanting.

Simply by heightening your awareness of who, where, and what you are, you alter your experience on every level.

The closer you get to the essential truth of who and what you are, the closer you get to *sat-chit-ananda*, or truth-consciousness-bliss, the ultimate goal of the yogi. If you are looking for happiness by fulfilling your desire to change the body, you may as well tune into the heavy metal station on the radio and wait for them to play Enya. You have to change the channel. When you tune into the very essence of what you are, you will find silence, and every answer to every question ever posed.

⊰ TUNING INTO YOUR ESSENCE ⊱

The body is the primary means to enlightenment.
—ancient Rishi sage

Close your eyes and feel your hands. How do you know they're there? You can't see them, but you can feel the energy that occupies them. Listen to that energy. That is what you are. Not the hands you see in the mirror, not the face you see in the mirror, but that energy. What separates your body from being a corpse? Vibration—life! Your thoughts and your body are animated by life force much the way an elaborate costume is animated by the dancer who wears it. When the dancer is gone, the costume is just a pile of fabric. In fifty or a hundred years, your hands and your face of flesh and blood will be nonexistent, but your energy is eternal.

So when you say, "I'm fat," that is an extremely limiting identification. Is that really what you are? Of course not, but it may be an identity you've bought into, and the more you buy into it, the more miserable you'll become. Seeking fulfillment in a thing as ephemeral as the human body is like running toward a mirage to get a drink. You reach the mirage, there's no oasis, and you're still thirsty. Let it go. The body may be an element of your experience, but it's definitely not the whole picture, and it won't change easily unless you drop your identification with it. Ramana Maharshi, a great yogi, said, "Abide as the Self." Abiding as the Self is like viewing your journey through the thick forest from the top of the highest tree. Your experience will be the most blissful if you can live in the simple awareness that you *are*—you exist, you are aware—without marrying your essence to mundane identifications like your shape and size. In your essence, you are not fat, out of shape, in shape, sexy, or not sexy. In your essence you are simply alive! You are!

And I can promise you this much, no matter how much you weigh, you are not fat. And neither am I.

⊰ **ASHTAVAKRA** ⊱

In India, there was a very well-known saint named Ashtavakra. In Sanskrit, the name Ashtavakra means "bent in eight places." When Ashtavakra was still in his mother's belly, his father, who was a very holy man, used to read to him from ancient scriptures. One day, while his father was reading, Ashtavakra interrupted him from his mother's womb (it happens in India) to tell him that his pronunciation was wrong, and asked if he would please correct himself. This made his father so angry that he put a very bad curse on Ashtavakra. He said, "When you are born, you will be deformed and bent in eight places."

The father then went to the king of the land to apply for a job as a holy man in the king's court. King Janaka did not like the father's discourse, so he condemned him to a life of austerities in the sea. Ashtavakra's father was forced to stand neck deep in the sea, practicing mantras and reciting scriptures all day, every day, for the rest of his life.

When Ashtavakra was born, he was indeed very deformed, and yet he was very wise. When he was eight years old, he went to King Janaka to ask for his father's release. Hunched over and limping because of his deformities, Ashtavakra entered the crowded hall of the palace where the king sat surrounded by his five hundred advisors. Peering down his nose doubtfully, one of the king's senior advisors asked, "Why have you come here?" Undaunted, Ashtavakra replied, "I've come to talk with the king," as he limped toward King Janaka. The room fell silent as the advisors stared at this crippled, crooked, little boy who could barely drag himself across the room, approaching the great, powerful king with such confidence. One by one, they all began laughing at him until the whole room was resounding like thunder with snickering and jeers. Ashtavakra also began to laugh, at first quietly, and then louder than anyone else in the room. Slowly, the advisors' laughter began to die down. One of them asked, "We know why we are laughing, but why are you also laughing?" Ashtavakra replied, "I am laughing because you all think that I am this body." With that, the room fell back into silence.

Ashtavakra addressed King Janaka, explaining that he had come to ask for his father's freedom from the austerities in the sea. The king considered Ashtavakra's request and told the crippled boy he would grant the freedom of his father if Ashtavakra could win spiritual debates with all of the king's advisors. King Janaka wrongly supposed that Ashtavakra would lose. To the king's surprise, Ashtavakra proved himself to be wiser and much more clever than each of the advisors. He won every debate, and he did it with such ease and brilliance that not only was his father freed, but Ashtavakra was appointed to the highest position in the king's court: the primary counselor.

It is said that Ashtavakra remained deformed for much of his life as a lesson to those who met him that there is more to existence than just the body. Later in his life, he healed his body and it was no longer crooked or bent.

In India, Ashtavakra is a historical figure, and his presence in the king's court and his written teachings remain evidence of his profound existence thousands of years ago. Here are a few quotes from the Ashtavakra Gita:

One who considers himself free is indeed free and one who considers himself bound remains bound. As one thinks so one becomes is a popular saying in this world, and it is true.

My child, you have long been trapped by body-consciousness. Sever the trap with the sword of knowledge "I am intelligence" and be happy.

I am not the body, nor is the body mine, I am intelligence itself.

Distaste for sense objects is liberation; love for sense objects is bondage. Such verily is Knowledge. Now do as you please.

Serene in practical life as well, the wise one sits happily, sleeps happily, moves happily, speaks happily, and eats happily.

Blessed indeed is that knower of Self, who, even though seeing, hearing, touching, smelling, or eating, is free from desire.

Light is my very nature and I am no other than that.

⊰ THE BODY IS MUTABLE ⊱

Now that you have one of the keys to existence—you are not your body—there is still a possibility that you are still experiencing yourself as a body. And even though you now know the essential yogic question of all time, "What am I?" you may still be pondering the essential question of our time: "Am I fat?"

Do you think that you're fat? Don't be shy. Most people feel fat some of the time. Some people feel fat all of the time. Many people are either on a diet, thinking they should go on a diet, beating themselves up for cheating on their diet, or even worse, thinking those around them should be on a diet.

I'm not exaggerating when I say that lots of people are so fixated on their physical appearance that it consumes most of their thought activity throughout the day. "Should I eat this?" "How do I look?" "I wonder how so-and-so thinks I look." "Do I look fat?" A huge amount of energy is poured into image awareness. Ironically, most people are so worried about what other people are thinking about them, they don't notice that their imagined observers are entertaining exactly the same self-conscious image obsession. Everyone is so intensely preoccupied with how they look, there's no energy left to look at anyone else. So, what's the point of worrying?

That said, according to the World Health Organization, obesity in the United States has reached epidemic levels. Nearly one third of the adult American population, about sixty million people, are considered obese, and yet most people's ideal physical condition is light, slender, and toned.

In general, there seems to be a Grand Canyon–sized disparity between how we want to be, how we think we should be, and what we are. And contained in this deep valley separating what we are and what we want to be is obsessive, intense, and senseless worry about body shape and size.

The body is changeable. Yogis have known this for thousands of years. But contrary to the current trend, yoga is not about, and has never been about, becoming a supermodel or a gymnast. Physical yoga is simply a means of perfecting the body and its functions to get it out of the way. The idea is to perfect the body in order to move past body obsessions and distractions, so that you are free to focus on deeper matters of existence. For example, getting sick and then spending mental and physical energy (not to mention a lot of money) attempting to heal yourself detracts from the energy that could be spent inquiring into the deeper nature of existence. As the body breaks down due to old age, or rough adulthood, time spent in physical agony or fear is time yogis would prefer to spend practicing yoga. As a result, the yogis developed ways to avoid these types of time- and energy-consuming body fixations. This might come as a big shock to you—especially if you currently worship at the altar of your local gym—but it is possible to perfect the body, maintain the body, enjoy the body, and stop worrying about it. The real yogis have been doing it for thousands of years.

⊰ FAT IS RELATIVE ⊱

Don't believe the hype.
—**Public Enemy**

◦─═◉═─◦

If you look beyond your immediate lifetime and examine the DNA you have accumulated from your ancestors, you may notice that the fashions of their times, and what they have set up your biology to expect in terms of body shape and size, is neither waifish, buff, nor athletic. Up until about forty-five years ago, thin was not in—ever. Thin meant you had a disease, you were starving because you were poor, or you just had that unlucky genetic trait that rendered you—as many grandparents might say—"skin and bones."

Being what we now consider unattractively fat has been, throughout most of history, a sign of fertility, prosperity, and the ability to survive. Before 1900, roundness in the belly was considered priceless protection against consumptive illnesses. For our ancestors, fat looked spankingly sexy on a prospective mate. Not-so-ancient Mae West and Marilyn Monroe would both be considered rather plump for a sex symbol by today's standards, but in their day, every curve was perfection. So, what happened?

The media is becoming exponentially more powerful, and at the same time, diets and health fads are proving to be highly profitable. It's big business for corporations to convince you that you have a serious problem and need to pay them to "fix" it. In our culture, we are bombarded by messages reinforcing the current trend in body shape and size. And that's all it is: a trend that has turned into a huge fear of fat. And as the yogis say, "What you fear will appear" and "What you resist will persist." According to the World Health Organization, just as the trend toward getting thinner really hit in the 1960s is when people began to balloon up like never before. And to many people's chagrin, we still seem to be inflating.

Are we so brainwashed as a society that we can't operate beyond the body images projected in magazines, television, movies, newspapers, and at grocery stores? Apparently so. It's like when you're being fed intravenously, and the clever nurse switches the liquid she's pumping into your body without moving the needle. You may not notice, especially if the nurse is well practiced and you're in a coma. What to do? It's time to wake up!

How do you wake up? Stop functioning based on the programming you have been exposed to. Think for yourself, and more importantly, *feel* for yourself. What is beautiful to you? Forget about how your body looks for a moment. How does it feel? It's your body. Why not decide for yourself how your body can be the best experience for you? Why not let go of trying to win everyone's approval or conform to a fashion? Why not just listen to your own insight? You are far more connected to your body and your body's needs than any cereal box, soda can, magazine, or weight-loss corporation.

Let go of wanting to look like someone else. You're not Hollywood's movie star flavor of the month. You're not this year's supermodel. You're you. Decide for yourself how you want to improve your experience of yourself. Don't worry about your audience or your critics. If you feel good, anyone who sees you will be drawn to you, no matter what your shape and size.

INNER YOGA

1. What is your sensory experience of your body? What preoccupies you? Do you have aches and pains? What feels good? How does your body move?

2. Take an inventory of physical characteristics you've wanted to change, and who you have lusted to look like (or unlike!). Make a list. Then go a step further and discern what kind of fulfillment and happiness you believe these changes will bring you.

 Is it possible for you to have fulfillment and happiness just as you are now? Imagine that you could take a shortcut and experience the fulfillment you think only someone shaped like a supermodel can have. Can you let go of needing to be something other than what you are? Just in this moment, let go.

3. Get out of a lacking frame of mind by focusing on what you have and what you are grateful for about your body. Make a list. Are you able to breathe? That's a plus. Are you able to walk? Do you have any fun with your body? From this appreciative frame of mind, you will have more access to immediate and lasting change—if you want it.

⊰ HOW TO CHANGE THE BODY ⊱

Most people would rather change their religion than change their diet.
—Dr. Roy Walford, *The Anti-Aging Plan*

⊷⊜⊶

If you can, imagine that your body is a pet. It's your responsibility to look after this pet, so you feed it, exercise it, and lovingly care for it. If you abuse this pet, it will misbehave. If you feed it the proper foods, exercise it, groom it, and let it rest, it will be the sweet emanation of joy and fun that it is inherently. You have to know a little bit about your pet so you can avoid potential disasters. It's well known that any animal who is fed foods that do not belong in its body—that have not been consumed by its genetic ancestors—will get sick. If you feed a dog enough chocolate, it will die. If you starve, then overfeed, then starve your pet, it will go a little nuts and may develop behavioral problems. Your body is like your dearest pet, and care and nurturing are essential if you want your experience of it to be easy and problem-free. The physical aspect of human existence is animal, and all the rules of nature apply. Just as you wouldn't knowingly abuse an animal, you must not knowingly abuse the body. The causes and effects of your actions, when you're dealing with the physical body, are obvious and clear. If you mistreat it, you will experience a reaction. It's necessary to free your thought process from the muddled messages seeping in from food commercials and societal norms if you have an interest in being free of the societal norm of disease and physical ailments. Become clear on what is good for the body.

Being acutely aware of one's behavior is one of the most simple wisdoms. The yogis say, "Wake up; don't be a sleepwalker." To begin to rouse from a life of deep sleepwalking is as simple as asking yourself, "What am I doing?" To knowingly consume cancer-causing substances and then act shocked when you're diagnosed with cancer is an example of unconscious behavior. To be rude and cruel to everyone you interact with and then be surprised when no one comes to your birthday party is acting unconsciously. To eat junk food constantly, then feel cheated when you feel—and look—junked out is a prime example of unconscious behavior. If you fail to exercise the body, neglect to feed it appropriately, forget to give it rest, and generally brush aside caring for it, what do you expect will happen? Perfecting the body isn't a matter of working a miracle, it's only a matter of being awake to your own behavior toward it.

"Fat" people—those whose shape and size compromises their well-being and makes them physically ill at ease—are fat for many reasons, mainly because they eat too much, and also because, well, they eat too much. Aside from a few physiological disorders and genetic predispositions, this is the main reason. What is too much? Consuming more calories than can be used by the body. Another primary reason is that "fat" people eat the wrong foods. The food is not inherently wrong—it might be good for some animal somewhere—it's simply not food fit to be consumed by a human body. Wrong foods include all the stuff that makes you fat, and I think you know exactly what I'm referring to: fatty meat, dairy products, cheeses, bakery products, gooey cookies, and unusual, unnatural, foul foods that are colorfully wrapped in crinkly plastic papers and have a shelf life of up to twenty years. You know, the good stuff (or so we're led to believe). Words to the wise: Just because it has a cool label and a funny commercial on television does not mean it won't make you fat, sick, or otherwise indisposed. Advertisements may promise that their product will give you confidence, friends, and everlasting joy, but what can I say? Don't believe the hype.

Just as you would be conscientious and take loving care of a fluffy little friend, you must be awake to the natural requirements of the body—if you don't want the body to be riddled with malice toward you, its keeper. Sustaining perfect physical health is simply a matter of transcending harmful programming and functioning in an alert, wakeful state instead of sleepwalking. Yogic wisdom demands conscious behavior, and this applies to food. Now that you know the most basic rules—(1) care for your body as well as your ability and knowledge permit and (2) feed it the appropriate human food in the right amount—you can begin consciously perfecting your physical health.

⊰ CHOOSE ⊱

Nine men in ten are suicides.
—**Benjamin Franklin, *Poor Richard's Almanack***

⊷⊷◉⊶⊶

The truth is that your experience of your body is for the most part up to you. Aside from diseases that are passed on genetically, you have an incredible amount of power to design your own shape, size, and physical experience. As you get conscious, it will be clear to you that there is a certain cause and effect involved in your behavior toward the body. In essence, you can choose whether you want to keep it in condition and make it last, or whether you want to let it wither away in poor health and end your experience in a physical body fairly soon. To a certain extent, the choice is yours.

For thousands of years yogis have been living well into their hundreds without any physical problems. They let go of the body when they consciously choose to. It has been done, it is possible, and it's never too late to begin.

Perfecting the body and extending the lifespan is worthwhile to the yogi because it allows the soul to stay on the planet and in a human body as long as possible. Experience in a body is precious and rare, because it is here that the soul has the greatest potential to realize freedom—if that is your intention.

"*Aturasya vikar prashamanamcha swasthyas swasthya rakshanam*" is easy to pronounce if you're a Sanskrit scholar. In case you can't understand Sanskrit, it was said by the yogis in India six thousand years ago and it means the following: "Eliminate diseases and dysfunction of the body, protect health, and prolong life." If you knew you could, wouldn't you?

INNER YOGA

1. Look around you at the people you see in your everyday life. From a nonjudgmental, objective point of view, what do you notice in their behavior toward food and their bodies? Are they conscious of what they're doing, or are they going through the motions of unconsciously programmed, sleepwalking behavior? Just notice what's going on around you.

2. Take a look at your day-to-day existence. How much of what you do is habit rather than conscious choice? Are you particularly attached to any unhealthy habits? Is adherence to the nutritional ideas of the media, your parents, and this culture working for you? Is it bringing you joy? Do you think you might be able to let go of some of the habits that don't bring you joy and well-being? Which ones? Make a list.

3. If you could let go of these habits and conditioning, would you? When?

⊰ YOGI FOOD: ANCIENT WISDOM AND MODERN KNOWLEDGE ⊱

Let your food be your medicine.
—**Hippocrates**

When I was about eighteen, I witnessed the slow and agonizing death of my grand-mother. She was a sweet, loving woman who, from as early as I can remember, baked rich, scrumptious cinnamon rolls, made candy from scratch, and the pastries—oh, decadent and delightful! Whenever I'd visit her, she'd give me anything I wanted. It was a festival of eating. My own mother didn't normally let me have sugar, so the taboo of it all was especially exciting. She loved me so much; she was always hugging and squeezing, laughing and playing like only grandmothers can. What can I say? I adored her. She ate a lot of rich, heavily sugared foods, and consequentially, she was a woman of biggish scope.

Eventually, she developed diabetes, and I witnessed the torturously slow demise of her health. She went from being a bright-eyed bundle of joy to a lethargic, moan-ing, hallucinating woman riddled with pain and ineffective painkillers. I watched her turn blue and sat by her hospital bed and held her hand as she slipped in and out of comas. Delirious and aching after much too slow of a physical descent, she eventually died.

If you've never seen someone in this much pain, I can testify that it's absolutely heart-wrenching. She became this ill not because she was a bad person, not because of her genes, not from a contagious bacteria, but from her diet and her diet alone.

I knew that this was not the way I wanted to die. This was more than enough to inspire me to go to every health seminar I could find. I began reading medical jour-nals and alternative health reports. I read every credible book on the subject of health and nutrition. I realized that ideally, eating is not a pastime or a hobby but a means of keeping the body free from pain and suffering. I met people who had, simply by changing their diet, cured themselves of diseases proclaimed incurable by doctors.

The yogic way is to perfect the body. At this time, with the combination of modern science, ancient wisdom, and one's own intuition, there's no reason to continue suf-fering with bodily complaints. The following section contains my suggestions, knowl-edge, and experience with regard to perfecting the body. It's my aim with these twelve points to help you achieve flawless health and longevity. If you're married to your habits and set in your ways, or if you like the idea of growing old in relentless pain, riddled with disease, by all means skip the rest of this chapter and get started on Rea-son 4. Even if you're not identified with your health at all—for example, if you do not experience yourself as a body, but just a floating cloud of bliss—you may still find something of value in the facts, statistics, and studies that will be an endless source of material for grossing out your friends and family while they're eating steak or inhaling Twinkies. I can only share with you what I know; what you do with it is completely in your hands.

As with any change in your diet or exercise regime, you should consult your doctor first. But make sure your doctor is up to speed with your personal needs and the latest breakthroughs in health and nutrition. For all of their years of training, most doctors only get about two weeks of diet and nutrition information, and most of that is how to deal with diabetics once they're already very sick. Although some doctors are rising to the occasion and broadening their horizons, many would rather play golf and remain under the thumb of large pharmaceutical companies than explore preventive health measures. I would recommend having a conversation with your family doctor to determine his or her degree of nutritional competence before taking any advice. If he or she does turn out to have mush between the ears and is uninterested in discussing nutrition—or just doesn't have time to actually have a conversation at all with you, the patient—then it's time to find a new, better, smarter doctor. Brilliant, compassionate, open-minded doctors do exist, so don't settle for less.

For yogis, the realization of enlightenment is the purpose of existence. Perfecting one's health is a means of eliminating painful distractions from this one-pointed quest. To the yogi, the realization of bliss in every moment is a good reason to prolong life and avoid physical suffering. The following twelve points have proven to be effective in maintaining great health in my life, and in the lives of many of my yoga students, who also follow these guidelines. They are points for perfecting physical health and are not meant to be used as material for further worry and suffering. I know lots of very happy, spiritual people who remain radiant and untroubled even though they eat what I would consider unhealthy diets. So, don't worry. If any of these points ring true for you, try them out. I'd recommend experimenting with how the application of these suggestions makes you feel. Notice how the body reacts and how you react. Always listen to your own intuition and do what seems best for your body.

1. AVOID SUGAR

According to a CSFII USDA survey, the average American consumes 20.5 teaspoons of granulated sugar a day. In one year, that adds up to 68.5 pounds per person. It is possible, however, to live a full, happy life without any extra sugar in it.

Sugar impacts the entire body physiology *dramatically*. A study of fifty married couples demonstrated conclusively that when sugar was removed from the diet, the number of arguments dropped 86 percent. Sugar produces wild mood fluctuations, fatigue, and irritability. Not only that, but it's highly addictive: Have you ever seen a child having a sugar jones? Angels turn into demons to get their fix.

It's not just sugar in its granular form that's habit causing, but some forms of certain carbohydrates that have a high glycemic index. If a food has a high glycemic index, it simply means that its sugars hit the body's systems quickly. Dr. Gabriel Cousens, author of *Depression Free for Life*, confirms that foods that have a high glycemic index cause wild swings in blood sugar, causing a high. That high is followed by a low, hypoglycemic state associated with tense mood, disinterest, depression, and an overall negative perception of the world. Some of the foods with the highest glycemic indexes are sugar, white bread and white flour products, processed fruit juice, white or instant rice, donuts, cookies, any alcoholic beverage, and rice cakes.

Food with high glycemic ratings will cause the most dramatic health swings, and these swings lead to dramatic health conditions. Instead of giving you a course in basic biology, I'll give you the explanation in a nutshell: Eating foods with lots of sugar (or high glycemic index) renders you insensitive to your own pancreatic insulin. This is like your TV becoming insensitive to the remote control; you can push buttons and hit the remote control against the couch, but the TV won't respond. Insulin is the hormone that opens the cell wall so blood sugar can get in. When you become insensitive to insulin, it's like your cell wall doorbell is broken. The insulin will show up with energy in the form of glucose, ringing the cell wall doorbell, but the door won't open. Thus, no matter how much food you shove through your body, energy won't get into your body's cells. And that is a major problem. As stated in the UK Prospective Diabetes Study, if you become insensitive to your own insulin, your body increasingly loses the ability to control blood sugar levels. Consuming foods with a high glycemic index often and regularly can send the body into a downward spiral of insulin insensitivity. First, the body overcompensates by producing lots of insulin to try to get glucose into the cells. Then the pancreatic cells get worn out and become unable to produce any insulin. Without insulin, the body can't regulate its own blood sugar levels. This is highly problematic and leads to obesity, depression, diabetes, and other undesirable conditions.

According to Dharma Singh Khalsa, M.D., founding member of the American Academy of Anti-Aging Medicine, stress itself increases cravings for high glycemic foods. Stress stimulates the production of cortisol, which in turn stimulates the release of a brain chemical, neuropeptide Y, that increases sugar cravings. If you satisfy your sugar craving by inhaling a candy bar or two, the body experiences more stress as it swings from a sugar high to a sugar low. Then you'll probably have another sugar craving.

Dr. Khalsa also warns that eating these high glycemic carbohydrates, like sugar, can actually damage your brain. Low blood sugar, often the result of the "sugar blues"—insulin insensitivity—can cause the permanent loss of brain neurons. Dr. Khalsa estimates that the normal person has lost millions of neurons—and memory power—just from blood sugar fluctuations.

The long-term effects of sugar are clearly illustrated when you compare the health of the French to that of Americans. Overall, the average French person eats four times the butter, smokes a lot more cigarettes, eats twice the animal fat, and eats three times the cheese that we do in the United States. Yet the French have substantially fewer incidences of heart disease, age-related illness, and other diseases conceptually linked to this type of decadent eating. Researchers have long been mystified by this seemingly incongruous miracle. Why are the French healthier than Americans when their diet is worse than ours? According to Dr. David G. Williams, one of the nation's leading authorities on natural healing, the answer lies in the fact that they eat one eighteenth the amount of sugar that the normal American eats. For every eighteen teaspoons of sugar that we eat, they eat only one.

Do yourself a favor and cut back your intake of sugar and other high glycemic foods as much as possible. Don't waste energy feeling guilty if you break down occasionally, but try to avoid it. Over time, you'll be happy to have your good health.

2. CUT OUT PROCESSED FOODS

A processed food is one that has been taken from its original state—for example, a fully formed potato just pulled from the countryside soil—and put through one or several processes. If processed instead of sold at the local farmer's market, this potato will likely be dehydrated at very high temperatures in a factory, then sent to a lab as flakes or a powder. At the lab, a chemical process will extract the starch from the powdered potato, heat it to 600°F, then put it in a can and sell it to an ice cream company. The ice cream company will hang on to it for a while, and somewhere between the time they put it into storage at their warehouse and the expiration date twenty years later (it doesn't last *forever*), they will put the potato starch in their ice cream along with some citric acid and who knows what other heavily processed ingredients. Sound yummy? That potato was processed, and the ice cream that the potato becomes a part of is also processed.

If you take a walk through the grocery store and actually read the ingredients of most of the items, you will find, for the most part, chemicals and substances derived from food that was fresh many, many years ago. Or, even scarier than that, you will find substances that were never fresh, but entirely synthesized in a lab. Most potato chips, breakfast cereals, anything BBQ flavored, hot chocolate powders, butter substitutes, jellies and jams, many breads, most crackers, and even many of those protein bars that pretend to be good for you are so intensely processed that the claims on the nutritive value column of their packaging may no longer be valid. Processed foods are essentially empty calories.

While your crackers and cheese-flavored spread in a tube might look pretty and safe, and may taste reminiscent of something that occurs outside of a laboratory, its twenty-year shelf life is an indication that it is intensely strange to put in your body. Take a moment and assess how you feel a little while after you've inhaled that adorably packaged cupcake designed to endure life on Mars. You might notice that it just doesn't do anything for you except satisfy the programmed idea that you've eaten something satisfying. Have you been brainwashed? If you have, how would you know? The hypnotized don't know they're hypnotized because, well, they've been hypnotized. But maybe somewhere in your heart of hearts, you just know.

Prana

In general, mankind, since the improvement of cookery,
eats twice as much as nature requires.
—Benjamin Franklin

⇥⊶⊷⇤

Processed foods are completely devoid of life force, which Indian yogis call prana, Chinese call Chi, Japanese call Qi, and Hawaiians call Mana. When you eat foods devoid of prana, you actually lose prana assimilating them. When you eat foods that are very fresh, you gain prana. If you stuff your body full of the cardboard junk that manufacturers try to pass off as human food, the lack of prana and nutrients not only leave you deficient, but rob you of what little life force you have left as the body tries to digest and survive the onslaught of chemicals. This causes you to be continuously hungry and possibly malnourished. You can eat tremendous amounts of food, be very overweight, and still feel and *be* starved! This is because your food is lifeless and nutrient taking instead of nutrient giving.

When you make the switch to very fresh foods, you will feel a boost in your energy. Because fresh food has more of its vitamins, minerals, and enzymes intact, you will not crave as much of it. When you begin to eat natural foods, your appetite actually drops on its own because your body's getting the life force and the nutrients it's designed for.

For thousands and thousands of years humanity has eaten natural whole foods. They didn't have a choice—it was natural food or starve. That's all there was until, in just the last one hundred years, industrialization, mass production, and the discovery of preservation techniques began tainting the nutritive value of the world's food supply.

According to Boyd Eaton, M.D., anthropologist at Emory University, 99.9 percent of our genes date back more than forty thousand years. Man was a prehistoric hunter gatherer who ate fruits, roots, tubers, nuts, seeds, herbs, vegetables, and, if the hunter was very lucky, whatever type of animal could be caught. That prehistoric man gene composition is more than 99 percent identical to primates—monkeys, gorillas, chimpanzees—who eat primarily grass, leaves, and berries. Genetically, our bodies are still programmed to receive nutrition in these ancient ways. Unfortunately, in our culture, it is the exception to find something to eat that hasn't been dry-cleaned, dehydrated, sprayed, canned, irradiated, oiled, fried, taken apart and coated in nitrogen, then re-assembled, shot up with hormones and/or antibiotics, or otherwise robbed of the natural nourishing qualities inherent in food. In the last hundred years, people have been getting sicker and sicker even as medicine has improved. Yet we don't seem to be noticing the association between our diet and our illnesses.

It's true that humans are highly adaptable and can survive on almost anything. But surviving doesn't mean that you won't be sick, in pain, uncomfortable, or depressed. Surviving only promises that you will have a pulse. The simple act of eating food that's ideal for the human body can give you a lifetime of physical ease, strength, and energy.

If you want to be healthy, it's important to eat what the human body is genetically designed to eat: real food from the earth—without much mileage between the farm and the dinner plate. So eat it! Pesticide-free natural foods are available at health food stores and even some mainstream grocery stores. Go straight to the produce section! Skip the boxed stuff, the canned stuff, the processed. Yes, natural organic foods can be a little more expensive. But when you calculate what you spend on healthy fresh foods and subtract it from what your hospital bill would have been after suffering a heart attack, liver disease, kidney failure, diabetes, pancreatitis, or who knows what else after a lifetime of eating junk food, you're actually saving yourself thousands and thousands of dollars.

3. EAT AS MUCH RAW FOOD AS POSSIBLE

Man is the only creature smart enough to cook his food, and dumb enough to eat it.
—Anonymous

This doesn't mean eat in the raw, although that can be fun, too. This means that as much as possible try to eat your food in its raw, uncooked, natural state. Why would anyone do this? Well, based on the knowledge that it is the primary concern of the yogi to increase life force through food, yoga postures, and right thinking, eating raw food is the obvious choice. Raw food has the highest life force, or prana, of any food. When you eat it, that force becomes one with you. This energy is nourishing, life giving instead of life taking, and in its purest form without any chemical, electrical, or industrial interference.

Enzymes

Approximately 85 percent of all vitamins and 100 percent of the enzymes are lost in the cooking process. If you cook anything above 118°F, the enzymes naturally found in that food are destroyed. The body needs enzymes to digest and assimilate nutrients in your food. Without the right enzymes, the body can't absorb vitamins or proteins. The bottom line: You can't get nourished without them. The pancreas makes enzymes, but your pancreas was designed by a genetic history of thousands of years of eating whole foods, most of which were raw. So the pancreas can only do so much if you're living off of coffee and microwaved popcorn (and I sincerely hope this is not your diet).

Undigested food particles left in the body can be really harmful—putrefying, fermenting, and becoming very toxic. Sometimes these particles enter the bloodstream to be cleansed, or they may cause gas, basically making you feel—and sometimes smell—like poop. Enzymes are crucial—for example, if the pancreas shuts down, the body dies.

If you're eating primarily cooked food, your pancreas has to work very hard to produce enough enzymes for your body to digest and even halfway assimilate what you eat. Getting all of your digestive enzymes from the pancreas is problematic because then the pancreas doesn't have the time or resources to do its other important job: produce metabolic enzymes. And that's a problem because you want your pancreas to supply you with as many metabolic enzymes as you can get! Metabolic enzymes basically make everything, *everything*, happen in our bodies. Without them, wounds can't heal, you age faster, you lose vitality, and you're less resilient against diseases, both genetic and contagious. Once an enzyme has done its job, it's destroyed, so the body needs a constant supply of fresh, helpful new ones.

When you eat raw foods, all of the enzymes your body needs to make the most of your meal are present *in the meal*. This allows your pancreas to supply you with more than enough metabolic enzymes, allowing for faster healing, more energy, less waste stored in the body, and countless other benefits. When you eat raw foods, the proof is in the raw pudding: Your energy increases, your clarity increases, your health improves, your weight greatly decreases along with your vulnerability to illness and disease.

Fire doesn't heal, it only destroys. When you subject any substance to fire, it eventually becomes pure ash—carbon. Current studies at UCLA, among other places, conclusively prove that carbon, when ingested, causes cancer. The more you cook your food, the worse the damage. Charred, barbecued, grilled, or any other method that blackens your food proves to be the most carcinogenic, according to these studies. If you must cook your food, steaming and slow cooking at low temperatures seems to be the least damaging.

Guilt Is Worse Than Being Enzyme Deficient

I've been mostly raw for thirty years. There have been times when I have experimented with eating cooked foods really just for the fun of it. The fun tends to be short-lived, though. There is a stark contrast in the way I feel when I eat cooked foods. It's nice to accept a piece of birthday cake and enjoy the taste of something familiar and comforting, but the pleasure only lasts for a split second, and then I feel a heaviness in my body. I get that toxic, icky feeling from eating something that's basically inedible. I always feel much better eating raw—lighter, cleaner, healthier, happier.

Even though I am totally devoted to eating raw, I don't recommend a 100 percent raw food diet for all people. Not because I don't think it would do them good—it would. However, you have to factor in our human tendencies. When transitioning to a raw diet, it's really common to be in a situation where the other people in your life become curious and often critical of the changes you're going through. Inevitably you want to fit in and so you chow down on some steamed rice and feel guilty. Who needs to feel guilty over having some rice?

If you eat as much raw food as you can—salads, fruits, nuts, smoothies—on a daily basis, that's wonderful. Some of the healthiest people I've ever met eat anywhere from 75 percent to 90 percent raw. The thing about eating a completely raw diet is that it seems that no matter which raw foods you eat, or how much of them, it's nearly impossible to gain excess weight. The abundance of enzymes keeps your body running so clean that it doesn't hold on to water weight, toxins, or extra fat. Those who eat 100 percent raw—no matter how much they eat—tend to be on the skinny side. Those who stay at 75 percent to 90 percent raw positively glow. When you eat raw foods, you're eating only nutrient-dense, easily assimilated, prana-filled food.

The Raw Yogi

For the yogi, raw food is great because it helps the flexibility of the body tremendously. Most raw foods have an extremely high water content. This not only helps keep the body hydrated (most people are chronically dehydrated), but it makes the body more flexible. At birth humans are 90 percent water, and as babies and children, we are more flexible, more resilient, and much cuter. A normal adult, however, is only about 60 percent water. If you're eating the Standard American Diet (SAD), you can expect your water content to continue to decrease as you age and your skin turns leathery and wrinkled. Physical degeneration is only natural if you're eating poorly and not doing all that you can for your body. Physical regeneration is natural if you assimilate lots of water, enzymes, nutrients, joy, and laughter. People living on whole, raw foods have been known to live to one hundred years of age, healthy and alert, and showing little or no sign of chronic degeneration.

A number of interesting experiments have been done with animals and raw food. Professor Robert Hartmann of the University of Berlin published a study in 1885 called "Anthropoid Apes." He fed several different kinds of primates (gorillas, chimps, and the like) the standard human diet at the time—boiled, baked, broiled, fried, and charred foods. These primates eventually developed a host of human ailments. They came down with coughs, colds, pneumonia, autoimmune disorders like cancer and psoriasis—all the diseases a human might develop. These diseases are not found in primates in the wild, nor did Hartmann's control group, who ate their normal diet of raw fruits, berries, and grasses, develop these illnesses.

In the 1940s, Dr. Francis Pottenger, a pioneer in nutrition and endocrinology, performed an experiment vividly illustrating the difference between eating a raw food and a cooked food diet. Studying about nine hundred cats over a ten-year period, he gave half of the cats raw milk and raw meat as a diet. He gave the other half the same milk and meat, but he cooked it. The results are astounding. The cats that ate the raw diet were healthy, with shiny coats and strong teeth and bones—physically sound in every way. The cats that ate the cooked diet experienced all of the diseases of modern man: leukemia, cancers, skeletal deformities, dental cavities, gum problems, arthritis, and so on.

As Pottenger carried the experiment over several generations, he discovered that the offspring of the raw food group continued to have excellent health, while the cooked food lineage degenerated more and more with each generation. The first kittens from the cooked food group were born sick and deformed, the second generation came out either riddled with disease or dead, and the surviving females of the third generation were completely unable to reproduce further. Pottenger's experiment is a simple illustration of how powerfully the food, and its relative rawness, can affect the body and its health.

Life begets life. No animal cooks its food. Though it's true that people have been cooking their food for a while now, how long do you think the body has been turning against itself with autoimmune disorders like cancer, lupus, and arthritis? Probably about as long as we've been cooking our food. And never before has our technology in the form of microwaves and other timesaving methods been so efficient at destroying foods' inherent nourishment. If you're thinking that eating raw food sounds fringe or weird, that's just your conditioning talking. If you look at it reasonably, you'll see that whatever walks this earth is meant to eat food from this earth as it is presented by nature. Try it. See for yourself.

If you're resistant to trying raw food, at least consider an enzyme supplement. Most people in the so-called civilized world, because of their diets and the diets of their parents, are completely enzyme deficient and would greatly benefit from taking enzyme supplements for the rest of their lives if they continue to eat cooked food.

4. CUT OUT ALL DAIRY

If you're the average American, you've been completely conditioned and brainwashed to believe that milk is a healthy food. And milk is a healthy food . . . for baby cows and only for baby cows. No other species drinks the milk from another animal species in the animal kingdom, and no other animal drinks milk after it's been weaned. It is not natural for a grown human to consume a substance that has been designed for a baby cow. Our bodies aren't genetically designed to process it. It certainly won't kill you instantly, but in the long run milk does have its drawbacks. Of course, if you are starving, living in a country struggling to survive a famine, or otherwise forced to sustain a pulse, it could be a viable alternative to death. But if you have a choice . . .

Free Drugs

First, let's take a look at the milk you buy at the grocery store. The cows that produced this milk are typically fed antibiotics, injected with hormones, and raised on extremely questionable feed. Every woman who's ever breast-fed knows that new mothers are advised not to consume alcohol or take certain medicines while lactating because the resulting milk will be tainted with it, damaging the baby. On the same note, when a cow is given megadoses of antibiotics, the antibiotics show up in the milk. That goes for the hormones and the questionable feed, too. So when you're drinking what you think is a wholesome glass of milk, you're really getting so much more for your dollar: free drugs!

Cows are fed hormones and steroids to make them larger and to produce more milk. This is enormously profitable for the milk companies and enormously harmful to your health. These hormones can and will affect you. Some effects include liver pollution, early-onset menopause, excess body hair, and early-onset puberty. BGH (bovine growth hormone) has been approved across the board by federal authorities and shows up in milk available at the market, but dairy farms aren't required to warn consumers of the possible risks associated with these hormones. According to Dr. Samuel Epstein, a leading cancer expert and professor at the University of Illinois, this hormone increases cancer of all kinds, especially breast cancer. Furthermore, the right combo of hormones and steroids can render a healthy grown man sterile.

In one of the more poorly thought out prevention methods, cows are also given antibiotics to stave off the rampant illness that afflicts most dairy farms. When consumed regularly by any animal—including a human being—antibiotics empower certain bacteria to become increasingly resilient. As the bacteria grow resilient to the antibiotics, the dairy farmers have to increase the cows' dosage. If you drink their milk, you're also taking their heavily dosed antibiotics. Bacteria in your body grows stronger, and you become vulnerable to serious illnesses. The next time you know-ingly take antibiotics, you might not feel their effect. The stuff in your milk could ac-tually be more potent.

Mutant Proteins

Let's just pretend that the cows are totally healthy and not drugged in any way. Re-gardless, all their nice healthy milk is pasteurized. The pasteurization process requires that the milk be heated to high temperatures to kill any bacteria that might have survived despite antibiotics. When a protein is heated, its molecular structure is altered. Amino acids become toxic when denatured molecularly, and as many see it, unfit for human consumption. Additionally, in yogic terms, the high heat has the effect of sucking all the prana from the milk. While the pasteurization process removes bacteria, it also destroys any benefits that might have been there to begin with. Pasteurized milk products—which include all the milk products you buy at the supermarket—are associated with allergies, heart disease, strokes, impaired circulation in many forms, digestive disturbances, sinus problems, earaches in children, lung problems including asthma, and more. Ac-cording to Dr. Neal Barnard, founder of the Physician's Committee for Responsible Medicine, Dr. Jonathan Wright, M.D., and Dr. Lane Lenard, Ph.D., experts on the sub-ject, men who avoid milk decrease the risk of developing prostate cancer substantially. And the prostate is something you generally want to hang on to.

If you're getting all of your protein from chugging down milk by the gallon, you may want to examine that habit. Does it do your body good, or does it feel good because you're used to it and it's comforting?

The Mucus Factor

Milk is extremely mucus forming. Although the body needs some natural mucus, you don't need as much as you probably have. Think of the last time you were run down with allergies or had a cold and you kept blowing your nose and coughing up mucus. Where did all this extra mucus come from? Unnaturally copious amounts of mucus come from undigested and indigestible dairy products. What's a little excess mucus among friends? Well, mucus can be dangerous. In excess it places crystal deposits on the walls of arteries and prevents healthy blood flow. These crystal deposits create an environment that can lead to joint pain, muscle aches, and inflammation.

Additionally, the presence of some of the constituents of milk, like casein, can actually turn mucus into more of a glue. Casein is actually a primary ingredient in some household glues. Milk, cheese, yogurt, ice cream, and the various other forms of cow milk can all act as a glue, gumming up your delicate, beautiful, fragile, circulatory, respiratory, and digestive systems.

A yoga student of mine had the most dramatic allergies. Every spring, throughout yoga class, he had to blow his nose about every five minutes. Talk about copious amounts of mucus—this guy had everyone else beat. I've never seen or heard so much mucus in my life. I suggested that he stop consuming dairy products for a few weeks to see if it might help. He did, and most of the symptoms of his allergies went away. He was so relieved. On top of that, without even trying, he lost about seven pounds he'd been trying to get rid of for several years but couldn't. He's still nondairy and doesn't miss the milk products—or the mucus—one bit. If you want to see remarkable weight loss, stop consuming all dairy products and the pounds will drop off you.

Cow milk does a body good, but only if you're a calf. Got milk? Got heart disease? Got arthritis? Got antibiotics? Got bovine hormones? Got mucus? Better to get conscious.

5. CUT BACK ON MEAT CONSUMPTION AS MUCH AS POSSIBLE

Without the killing of living beings, meat cannot be made available, and because killing is contrary to the principles of ahimsa,* one must give up eating meat.
—**The Laws of Manu, sacred yogic text**

‹‹═◉═›•

* Ahimsa is an ancient yogic term that translates from the Sanskrit to mean "harmlessness." "Having no ill feeling for any living being, in all manners possible and for all times . . . should be the desired goal of all seekers" is a passage also from The Laws of Manu.

You and Meat

Before I get into the deep, ancient stuff, let's talk about you and what meat can do to you. In study after study, meat has been linked to heart disease, obesity, diabetes, and several forms of cancer. If you eat meat three to four times a week, you have three to four times the risk of developing colon cancer compared to those who rarely or never eat it.

There was a time when meat was very pure. Herded animals and fowl lived their lives in a natural environment, ate foods that came directly from the earth, and lived with clean air and water. That time is over. The meat sold in supermarkets comes from animals raised in tiny cubicles, often unable to take a step. They are fed the cheapest food possible: highly processed feed that sometimes includes ground animal parts that don't sell well, like brains, hooves, beaks, and the like. Cows don't naturally eat other cows. A pig wouldn't eat another pig in the wild. Cannibalism can lead to serious illnesses, like mad cow disease.

These animals are routinely injected with antibiotics to prevent infections, steroids to accelerate growth (so they can be killed sooner), and hormones to make them bigger. These substances don't have a chance to be cleansed from the animals' bodies since the animals don't exercise, get enough fresh water, or eat pure foods. Where do you think these substances go when the animal is slaughtered and then cooked? Nowhere. The hormones, antibiotics, and steroids stay right there in the muscle tissue—the meat that you eat. Think you're getting a good price on some pork loin? Think again. You're getting so much more.

And there's more. When an animal is killed—either by decapitation in a slaughter line, by strangulation, or by lethal injection—its tissues continue to live for many hours after it's technically dead. The cells and tissues keep on excreting toxic waste the way they always have, and usually the toxin load is immense in animals raised for consumption. But there's a glitch: The animal's circulatory system is no longer pumping blood or oxygen through the body to remove these toxins. The arteries keep contracting, pushing now waste-laden blood into the tissues that you might later serve on a sesame seed bun for dinner. If you're not already feeling sick, this should push you over the edge: If there was some process to remove toxins from the meat (there isn't), the meat would be pure and . . . there would be no taste. According to Peter Ragnar, noted naturopath and biologist, meat's flavor comes from cellular waste that, given the opportunity, would have been flushed from the animal's system and eliminated in the natural way—through its organs, then urine and feces. It's would-be poop. So what are you really ingesting when you eat meat? You do the math.

There's something else in your meat that no one is telling you about: fear. Animals know when they're about to die. They feel the fear of the animal ahead of them in the slaughter line. As a natural response to this fear, the animal's body shoots adrenaline through its system, and then it's killed. That adrenaline has nowhere to go. It stays in the tissues, so when you consume the meat of a slaughtered animal, you literally consume the fear and the violence of the animal's death, still intact in chemical form in the tissues. If you're just not sure about all of this, see what happens to your anxiety levels, your stress levels, and your mood swings when you cut back or cut out meat.

Your Body and Meat

Even if meat wasn't poison to begin with, which it seems to be these days, our bodies turn meat into poison anyway, making it doubly deadly. If you have pointy claws that retract and a furry tail, this may not apply to you. But if you are like most human beings, your body is built to be a vegetarian. To begin with, our digestive tract is four times longer than a meat eater's. Rib eye lovers might say, so what? Well, by the time meat gets to a place where it can be digested, it has already started to rot. Our gastric fluids don't have the antiseptic and germicidal properties available in the digestive fluids of a carnivore, and the meat has to travel four times the distance. So what you are sending into your system is putrid, rotting meat—also depleting your enzyme supply.

It's like driving two hundred gallons of raspberry sherbet in an open bed pickup truck four hundred miles on a hot summer day. By the time you reach your destination, it will not only have melted, it will have turned rancid. Our intestinal system is like that long drive and open bed pickup. What you need is what dogs and other carnivores have—a ten-mile drive and a freezer truck. Their load will arrive intact and ready for assimilation.

We have smaller livers than carnivores, we produce less bile, our kidneys can't handle the excess uric acid—which leads to gout and kidney disease—and our saliva is alkaline as opposed to acidic, like that of a carnivore. Once you swallow meat, it enters your system and begins to rot immediately. The body will do its best to assimilate it, but digesting meat often takes more out of you than you realize. If you do eventually get it out of you via some time on the toilet, the smell will probably make you famous in any frat house.

What doesn't get digested—many times almost half—festers in your colon, causing ammonia to build up around the rotting meat. This rotting stuff does about as much for your organs as a spoonful of shattered glass. Meat can get stuck in the twists and turns of our long digestive tubes for years, and a few years is often just the right amount of time for a serious disease to develop. The lining of your colon can grow around the stuck meat and ammonia, turning it into a time bomb. Noxious waste can leak into your system through this lining, slowly poisoning you. During autopsies, it's not uncommon to find upward of fifty pounds of mucus, stony fecal matter, and lumps of undigested meat. The bottom line: Our bodies aren't equipped to deal with meat without developing a disease as a by-product.

Some people have said they feel more energized when they eat meat, and ask me how they could feel energized if it's such nasty stuff. Meat is very acidic, as well as being toxic. Your body reacts to the acidity and the adrenaline in the meat, and for a little while, it has a stimulating effect on your nervous system. But, like coffee, this is a temporary physical response, which later turns into lethargy. The adrenaline lasts for a few minutes, but the poisons can stay with you for a long, long time.

Meat eaters might not be able to smell each other—just like smokers can't usually smell other smokers—but vegetarians can almost always smell a meat eater immediately. I don't want to make anyone self-conscious, but it's not a sexy smell, it's not a cute smell, it's not even a friendly smell. It's kind of a rot odor. It's distinctive. Even if meat weren't poison and didn't turn into poison in the body, the smell alone is reason enough to let it go.

Chicken

Yes, chicken is also meat, and everything stated in the preceding meat section applies to chicken and other fowl. But I'd like to point out a few seldom mentioned facts about the current condition of chicken sold in supermarkets and restaurants. Due to the inhumane diet (often ground chicken) and conditions in which chickens are raised before they're killed, they seem to be developing chicken cancer at an alarming rate. According to Dr. Virginia Livingston-Wheeler, "Most of the chickens on the dining tables and barbecue grills of America today have the pathological form of PC (Progenitor Cryprocides) microbe." She proposes that this chicken cancer may be transmissible as a virus to human beings upon consumption. She contends that most of the chickens packaged for human ingestion have tumors visible to the eye, but because of the rushed production, they slip past the inspectors. Nobel Prize winner and researcher at the Rockefeller Institute for Medical Research, Dr. Peyton Rous, contends that 95 percent of the chickens sold in New York City are certainly cancerous. He concurs with other researchers that this chicken cancer may be transmissible. Is your fried chicken really fried cancer tissue? It's certainly worth consideration.

Fish

I know many "vegetarians" who also eat fish. But the sad, scientific truth is that fish is not technically a vegetable. The argument for including fish in the diet is usually for the health benefits. Unfortunately, presuming that eating fish will do anything for your health is a couple of centuries out of date.

If the world's oceans and rivers were as clean as they were two hundred years ago, fish could be beneficial for your health. These days, you have two choices: farmed fish and fish caught in the wild. The world is a big place, and fish caught in the wild could come from anywhere—possibly from a toxic dumping site in a country without strong pollution policies (there are many), or from an area that has high levels of heavy metal pollution, or worse, from an area with biochemical hazardous wastes. Many fish— especially canned tuna—contain higher levels of mercury and other toxic substances than government agencies would ever allow to remain in drinking water. Eating fish is like playing Russian roulette—very risky.

Your second choice is farmed fish. They live by the thousands in little pools and are just scooped out to be sold. Seems like a good idea economically, but there are serious problems, not the least of which is keeping the water clean. Most farmed fish have a high enough ammonia content from ingesting fish urine that you could effectively use them to mop your floor. But I wouldn't eat them.

The CSPI (Center for Science in the Public Interest) has been petitioning the FDA (Food and Drug Administration) for some time now to test fish for potentially life-threatening substances. The CSPI has taken a firm stance, warning that fish currently on the market contain high levels of hazardous bacteria, as well as ammonia, toxic heavy metals, and various dangerous and identifiable industrial pollutants. But there are so many fish in the sea—to test each one is time-consuming and labor-intensive.

Wild fish naturally contain high levels of omega-3 fats, which are very good for you if they're uncooked. If you heat these fats, they become rancid, toxic, and cancer causing. If you eat the fish raw, you'll get the omega-3s, but you'll probably get much more. There's a good chance you'll pick up microscopic parasites—especially from salmon—which can live in the body undetected for thirty years or more, breeding more parasites, depleting your body of vitamins and minerals, and causing horrible body odor, depression, bad breath, and stomach problems. Even if fish were a vegetable—and it's not—it doesn't do you much good.

Still think you're a meat eater? If you stop eating meat, you may go through withdrawal and crave it. But rest assured that it's not because your body needs it, but because you're addicted to the drugs and the adrenaline in the meat. Look at it this way: If you're driving down the road and see an animal that's been hit by a car, or a cow grazing in a pasture, or a chicken running around, do you salivate? Do you have passionate, violent, but enjoyable thoughts about ripping it apart and eating it? How about when you see or smell a perfectly plump, ripe peach hanging from a tree? Or fresh, sweet blueberries hanging from a bush? Do you salivate then?

Yoga and Meat

The wanton destruction of life is against the true nature of the heart.
—**Peter Ragnar,** *How Long Do You Choose to Live?*

◦─◦◎◦─◦

Yogis have their own reasons for abstaining from meat. Yogis don't always look for nourishment first; rather, they look at the vibration of the food. When I say *vibration*, I'm referring to the source of the food, and the attitude and intention of the person preparing it. First, yogis consider the growers of the food. Are the farmers full of gratitude and love, and do they enjoy growing food, or are they angry and filled with hate for their job and all vegetables? These farmers handle the food, and the yogis believe that their feelings, or vibration, go into the food and thus go into your body if you eat it. Next, yogis consider the cook. Is the cook full of love and good intention, or full of resentment and anger? Yogis have experienced that the attitude of the cook produces energy that affects the vibration of the food, and that food can be poisoned by a bitter cook. Yogis often choose to add their own vibration to food before eating it in the form of prayer, blessings, or any other method of energetic cleansing—a very good idea!

The most essential aspect of eating food with a good vibration, or high vibration, is to not associate violence with what you put into your body. The general rule of thumb here is don't eat anything that had a face. Yogis believe that animals possess consciousness, therefore to kill them and eat them is to put the energy of fear and violence in the body, because that is the emotional experience of the animal as it dies.

If, like the yogis, your aim is to be peaceful and happy, you won't want to cause harm to a sweet, kind, sensitive being with feelings. If you don't believe that animals have feelings, step on your dog's foot and see what happens. Animals express fear, playfulness, love, helpfulness, and a range of other emotions. If you raise an animal from the time it is born, and you play with it, look after it, and get to know it, it would be nearly impossible for you to kill it and eat it. Why? Because animals possess consciousness. The corpse of a being that's led a life of abuse capped off with a violent, horrible death—the meat you find at the grocery store—is the last thing you want to ingest. Why pollute your body with fear and violence if you don't have to? There are other options.

That's why yogis recommend vegetarianism. Many of these vegetable-loving yogis live to be between 100 and 120 without physical problems and wrinkles, but with lots of big smiles.

If you live in a place where you don't have access to fruits and vegetables like in some parts of Tibet or the North Pole, it's a different story: You are eating what is available in order to keep your body alive. When you live in most parts of the United States, however, where you can choose from a million different life-sustaining nutritious foods, it is neither optimum nor necessary to eat an animal.

I personally know, and know of, many people who have felt much calmer, healthier, and happier simply by the adoption of a vegetarian diet. But even if you can't see yourself instantly incorporating all of the vegetarian suggestions I make for the modern yogi, even one adjustment can give you some perspective on the power the diet has over the physical body. Often even the slightest improvement of one's day-to-day existence has resounding repercussions. Dick Gregory, a famous comedian in the 1960s and 1970s, drank a fifth of Scotch whisky and smoked at least a pack of cigarettes every day. He was a large, large man—rotund, grand in the belly, heavyset, full-bodied—you get the idea. He suffered from an ulcer and serious migraine headaches. One day, he decided to stop eating red meat. He came to this decision on his own; he just had a strong feeling that it wasn't doing him any good. Despite drinking the same amount and continuing to smoke, Dick Gregory experienced profound changes in his health simply from the absence of red meat. His body went from being enormous and pot-bellied to slender and lean. His ulcer and migraines went away.

How to Go on Living Without Meat

Most people eat meat because they think they need it for protein, but you don't need as much protein as you might think. In fact, you could be getting too much. Yes, you can get too much protein. How much is too much? According to the World Health Organization, Americans consume primarily meat-derived protein—upward of one hundred grams of protein each day, which is way too much. According to Dr. Gabriel Cousens, the average American eats two hundred pounds of meat each year. Accounting for average life expectancy, that translates to about 11 cows, 1 calf, 3 lambs, 23 hogs, 45 turkeys, 1,100 chickens, and 826 pounds of fish in one lifetime.

Too much protein will clog your system and can lead to several diseases. According to Dr. Paavo Airola, author of *How to Get Well* and one of the world's most respected nutritionists, high protein diets can lead to arthritis, pyorrhea, schizophrenia, atherosclerosis, heart disease, cancer, kidney damage, premature aging, and, most frequently, osteoporosis. It's well known among nutrition experts that if protein levels are in excess of the body's needs, the body becomes acidic, which is contrary to its natural, healthy state. To counteract this acidity, the body will pull calcium from the bones, resulting in higher incidences of osteoporosis in women who maintain high protein diets. According to the *Journal of Clinical Nutrition*, female vegetarians have five times less bone loss than high protein, meat-eating women. Additionally, high protein diets derived primarily from meat are extremely high in phosphorous, which also draws calcium from the bones, resulting in loss of bone density. Regardless of how much calcium you take as a nutritional supplement, if the body is too acidic or full of phosphorous, the bones won't be able to hang on to it.

The World Health Organization suggests thirty-two grams of protein each day, the *Journal of Clinical Nutrition* suggests between twenty and thirty-five grams, and everyone agrees that protein is safer and easier to assimilate if it's not derived from an animal source. I recommend anywhere between twenty and forty grams a day, depending on your lifestyle and individual need. There are a couple of fad diets out there that recommend consuming superhigh doses of protein and eliminating carbohydrates. This is certainly not the safest thing to do, especially for extended periods of time, as high protein slows down the production and release of insulin, which stores amino acids and regulates blood sugar. Throwing your insulin off this way can result in certain types of diabetes. These high protein diets have been recycled about every ten years since the sixties—remember the no bread diet? Inevitably, the inventor of the diet advertises and merchandises and sells and sells until he is as rich as he can get and then retires. Yet, as a whole, the American population gets more and more obese and diseased. Percentages of obesity climb dramatically as the years go by. Look at the people who recommend extremely high protein diets. Do they look radiant, youthful, and joyful, or do they radiate a dull density? You decide.

You can get more than enough protein from a diet of fruits, vegetables, nuts, and whole grains. There are also great protein powders available that are made from brown rice and not heat processed. Therefore they retain most of their prana (life force), nutritional value, enzymes, and the original, pristine amino acids.

6. EAT THE GOOD FATS

Fat-Free Is Silly

The fat-free fad that swept the world is a great example of the inevitable dumbness of broad generalizations about diet. The fat issue simply isn't black and white. Fatty acid metabolism is a very important process in your body. If you're not getting any omega-3 fatty acids, the result could be depression, psoriasis, asthma, rheumatoid arthritis, and many other unpleasant and distracting ailments. Omega-3s have been proven effective in regulating heart arrhythmia, lowering triglycerides, normalizing high blood pressure, improving focus and concentration, alleviating symptoms of depression, easing rheumatoid arthritis pain, improving irritable bowel syndrome, controlling insulin levels in type 2 diabetes, decreasing the symptoms of asthma and COPD, preventing cancer, and reducing general pain and inflammation. They will also do wonders for your hair and skin. Omega-3s are found in small amounts in sea weed and dark leafy greens, and in more substantial quantities in flax seeds/oil, hemp seeds/oil, and pumpkin seeds/oil.

According to cardiologist Dr. Stephen Sinatra, a fellow of the American College of Cardiology and the American College of Nutrition, omega-3s benefit every tissue in the body. According to the *American Journal of Medicine*, in clinical trials involving more than fifteen thousand patients, omega-3s were shown to reduce fatal heart attacks.

Omega-6 fatty acids are equally great for the body when combined with omega-3s. Omega-6s are found in almonds, sesame seeds, sunflower seeds, olive oil, canola oil, safflower oil, sunflower oil, fish oil and fat, and soy products. By themselves, omega-6 fatty acids aren't so great for you. The average American gets too much of them. But if you combine omega-6s with omega-3s in just the right proportions, the results are amazing and very conducive to good health.

You should have anywhere from between one part omega-6 to every two to four parts omega-3s. This combination prevents inflammation, which over the long term helps to prevent heart disease and other chronic ailments. All by themselves, walnuts have the perfect balance of omega-3s and omega-6s.

You can make delicious salad dressings out of a base of raw tahini (sesame seeds and flax oil. Add a little lemon and whatever else suits your taste, and your fatty acid requirements will be satisfied.

If You Must Cook with Fat . . .

It is important not to heat essential fatty acids. According to Dr. Sinatra, oxidation—which the heating process speeds up—transforms omega-3s into a rancid, toxic substance. People often turn to fish for omega-3s, but it's a risky thing to do because these oils go bad if they're exposed to even a little light, let alone a skillet. So be careful. Better to go for the raw vegetable sources if you're looking for any health benefit. The same goes for omega-6s: When heated, this essential fatty acid mutates into a carcinogenic state. So, don't cook with these oils!

If you're going to cook with an oil, it's much better to use a saturated fat, which won't become carcinogenic when exposed to heat. Saturated fats are solid at room temperature and turn to liquid when you heat them. Coconut butter is by far the best fat to cook with.

The Bad Fats

If your aim is to remove potentially life-threatening illnesses from your list of things to worry about, a good rule of thumb at the supermarket is to avoid hydrogenated and partially hydrogenated fats. These guys are toxic, toxic, toxic, and they're in just about everything that's processed. Mayonnaise, potato chips, those packaged cakes and cookies, even some of the packaged food that claims to be healthy are loaded with hydrogenated fats.

To make a fat hydrogenated, processors must inject and bubble in hydrogen. The hydrogen is valuable to profit margins because it makes the fat last almost forever. Baked stuff, fried snacks, fish sticks, frozen french fries, some peanut butters, lots of butter substitutes like margarine, some butters, microwave popcorn, pancake mixes, salad dressings, some ice cream and soy ice creams, many cheeses, and even some soy cheeses are loaded with hydrogenated fats. Anything with the word *hydrogenated* or *partially hydrogenated* in the ingredient list is bad, bad news. Roughly 75 percent of the Standard American Diet (SAD) contains hydrogenated fats, so stay very, very alert, especially if you're a standard American.

What can hydrogenated fats do to you? Increase free radical damage to cell membranes. And what does that mean for your health? Free radical damage speeds up the aging process, causes internal inflammation—which leads to hundreds of other serious conditions—creates enzyme deficiency, and can lead to cancer. To eat it is to self-destruct: You may as well light yourself on fire while you're eating this stuff (don't really ignite yourself—I'm just making a point). But you will save yourself a lot of heartache and anxiety simply by avoiding hydrogenated fats.

7. MAINTAIN AN ALKALINE BODY

All decay, degeneration, and disease occur in highly acidic states. The body's optimal state is one of alkalinity. Hazel Parcels, N.D., a professional nurse who lived 106 healthy years, was a pioneer in the discovery of the pH level's effect on the body. She nearly died in 1929 when she was diagnosed with incurable tuberculosis, with kidney and heart complications. She was forty years old, and her doctors sent her home to die. She cured herself by becoming a master of what she called "kitchen chemistry"— eating foods that encourage physical alkalinity. She didn't die at the age of forty, as her doctors had expected. A beautiful, vibrant woman with a radiant complexion and an unfettered joy for life, she died peacefully at the age of 106.

Stationery companies advertise acid-free paper because it lasts several hundred years, as opposed to acidic paper, which deteriorates rapidly. Paper doesn't have the life force flowing through it that you do, so imagine what is possible for you if you alkalize your body. If you put a cancerous tumor in a container full of an alkaline solution, it will dissolve in three hours. On the other hand, if your saliva is very acidic, your teeth could rot and fall out in a comparable amount of time.

In the human body, alkalinity is conducive to health and acidity is conducive to disease. There are certain functions of the body that must be acidic—primarily digestion—but overall the body craves an alkaline state. When healthy babies are born, they are in an alkaline state. As we grow and pollute the body with impure foods, negative thoughts and experiences, shallow breathing from stress, and chronic dehydration, the body slowly becomes more and more acidic.

There are several things you can do to return the body to its natural, perfectly balanced alkaline state. First and foremost, BREATHE! The next time you are stressed out, running errands, or stuck in traffic, notice your breath. Do you even breathe at all? It is common to get into the habit of taking short, shallow breaths when you're frightened or even mildly anxious. What happens right before the climactic explosion in any action film? You hold your breath because you're afraid. Along with sending a message to the body that it's in danger, shooting adrenaline into your tissues, and causing the muscles to tense up, stress and fear cause you to take in less oxygen and let go of less carbon dioxide.

Breathe deeply right now. Just breathing can take you from a state of fear into an open state of peace and well-being. Regular deep breathing regulates the heartbeat and calms the mind. Just breathing helps prevent disease, aging, and depression. And long, slow, deep breaths alkalize your body more effectively than anything else. Fresh, raw fruits and vegetables and their juices are also powerful alkalizers. Although some raw foods are acidic before you eat them—like lemons—your body's reaction to their assimilation is alkaline.

Also, try to stay in a positive state of mind. Ever notice that when you get angry or really negative, your breath gets worse and your body odor more offensive? If you haven't, those who are close to you have noticed it, and they've asked me to mention it to you. That's your body becoming acidic. So develop a sense of humor if you don't already have one—it could save your life.

You can test your body's pH by spitting on a pH test strip (available at most drugstores) several times throughout the day. You may as well try it because spitting on paper and watching it change colors is fun, even if you're not that interested in improving your health.

8. DRINK WATER

According to *Health Science* magazine, at least 75 percent of all Americans are chronically dehydrated. In most people, what is actually thirst is misinterpreted as hunger.

So you eat and eat, never feeling satisfied, because you're actually thirsty. Or worse, you drink soda pop or some other processed product of industry that is full of sodium (among other things). This works as well to quench your thirst as throwing kerosene on a raging bonfire effectively extinguishes the flame. Even worse for you than canned, carbonated, or chemical-rich consumable products of industry, caffeine and alcohol effectively shut off vasopressin, a pituitary hormone that maintains your body's hydration and memory. So drinking caffeine, alcohol, soda pop, or other strange forms of processed liquid to quench your thirst is like trying to drive a car forward with the gear stuck in reverse: It doesn't work.

Your normal thirst is not really an accurate indicator of your level of hydration. By the time you notice you're thirsty, you're already very dehydrated. Lack of water in your body, which is ideally 60 to 70 percent water, causes decreased flexibility, water weight gain, difficulty focusing, memory damage, wrinkling and other signs of premature aging, constipation, compulsive eating, and much, much more. Drinking plenty of water is like giving your internal organs a refreshing shower. Water prevents many diseases simply by keeping your system free of waste, so drink as much water as you can, unless you enjoy wrinkles and long hospital stays.

When it comes to water, the wetter the better. If you don't know what wet water is, you're missing out. Wet water has a lower surface tension and less viscosity, making it easier for the body to absorb. Do you ever feel like water goes straight through you without hydrating you? That's because it does. Water with high surface tension can't get into your cells—its molecule clusters are too big. Wet water has a high concentration of small clusters of water molecules. It's absorbed by the aquaporin channels in your cells more effectively than less slippery waters. Aquaporins were recently discovered by researchers at Johns Hopkins University as the water-bearing protein channels in the cell membrane that manage the flow of pure water into the body.

You can taste the difference between wet water and normal water; wet water is more slippery tasting, easier to swallow, and almost tastes sweet. Wet water feels wet because it is microclustered, and physiologically finds its way into your body with more ease, hydrating you more completely.

It is important to drink water that's as pure as possible. Bottled water is expensive and unreliable, so I recommend investing in a high-quality reverse osmosis water purification system that you can hook up in your own home. You can also find filters that enhance the microclustering of water. As a side note, tap water is filled with chlorine and industrial pollutants that will get absorbed through your skin, especially in a hot shower, so a shower filter is also a sound investment in your health.

Finally, it's better to drink water between meals rather than with meals. Loading up on water while you're eating is pouring water on healthy digestive fire. Water dilutes the acid in your stomach, making it very difficult to digest food properly, resulting in bloating, gas, or undigested food left in your system. It's best to do one at a time: Either eat or drink, but don't do both simultaneously.

9. RESTRICT YOUR CALORIE INTAKE

As houses well stored with provisions are likely to be full of mice,
so the bodies who eat too much are full of diseases.
—Diogenes

The Japanese district of Okinawa has the greatest percentage of people living past the age of one hundred ever reliably documented and the longest average life expectancy in the world. Okinawans eat nutrient-dense food, but they happen to eat 17 percent less food overall than the Japanese average and 40 percent less than the American average. The Okinawa Centenarian Study, presented at the annual meeting of the American Geriatrics Society, found that Okinawan elders, compared to Americans, are 75 percent more likely to retain cognitive ability, get 80 percent fewer breast and prostate cancers, get 50 percent fewer ovarian and colon cancers, have 50 percent fewer hip fractures, and have 80 percent fewer heart attacks. The researchers who conducted this study credited the Okinawans' longevity and good health to their diet, which was consistently low in calories but rich in nutritive value.

It's been suspected for a long time that caloric restriction has some health benefits, but it wasn't until Dr. Roy Walford and some of his colleagues did a massive study on the subject, called Biosphere 2, that reliable scientific evidence proved that calorie restriction not only creates better overall health, but slows biological aging and increases life expectancy. This human experiment started the ball rolling, and ever since, mounting evidence—like the Okinawa study—has pointed toward the numerous advantages of calorie restriction.

Calorie restriction does not mean anorexia or malnourishment, both of which shorten life and damage the body. It means smaller portions of intensely nourishing foods. This approach works for the body in many ways: The body doesn't have to deal with empty calories, excess fat slowing down the system, or processing the tremendous amount of waste most people push through themselves on a daily basis. Those who practice calorie restriction are thinner, live longer, and have less incidence of disease.

Calorie restriction is the only known way to extend the life span and enhance health in all species. As reported by the *American Journal of Physiology* and the *Journal of Gerontology*, among many others, by reducing their normal caloric intake by half, animals have lived twice as long as their normal projected life spans, with less disease and more effective immune systems than their peers.

In a continuing study being done in the city of Baltimore, researchers have identified certain biological markers that occur in men who are living the longest. Lower temperature, lower insulin levels, and a steady amount of the hormone DHEAS are the common factors in these healthy elderly men. A study being done by the National Institute on Aging, led by researcher George S. Roth, has found that laboratory animals placed on a calorie-restricted diet live 40 percent longer lives than their peers, and these animals share the same biological markers as the Baltimore humans. This can be translated to mean that a human on a calorie-restricted diet could live 40 percent longer than the normal projected life expectancy. So instead of living until 80, you could live upward of 112—in great health. Not only does calorie restriction increase life span, but it seems to slow biological aging so that an eighty-year-old looks and feels more like a fifty-year-old, and a forty-year-old looks and feels more like a twenty-year-old. According to Dr. Roy Walford, the foremost authority on the subject, it's important to reduce your caloric intake gradually while intensifying the nutritive value of what you eat.

Yogis have always practiced eating only what the body requires and nothing more. Part of this practice has to do with keeping the body supple and sensitive. A true yogi's main concern is reaching a transcendental consciousness—or enlightenment—

through yoga and other practices, including meditation. Anyone who's tried to meditate, practice yoga, or even pray on a full stomach quickly realizes that it just doesn't work very well. The prana (life force) is so involved in digesting food, it doesn't go up into the higher chakras. You're more likely to pass out or take a nap than you are to reach a heightened state of awareness. A lot of heavy food can be slightly numbing—the opposite of the yogi's pursuit of sensitivity, truth, and life.

A long life without the distraction of disease is a universally welcome condition. Yogis have known for ages that eating less lengthens life, and the longer a yogi has to live, the longer a yogi has to pursue the experience of the ultimate reality. Yogis also aspire to prevent disease and the tendency to replace the sustaining energy of a higher power with food (food addiction). These distractions detract from more spiritual endeavors.

If you'd rather eat buckets of nonnutritious food than live a healthy, long life, go ahead. It really is up to you. But it's important to know that you do have a choice.

10. FAST

From hunger I saw one man die, from eating I've seen hundreds die.
—Benjamin Franklin

--->==◉=<---

For thousands of years, yogis have fasted to purify the body, strengthen the will, and feed the soul. Abstaining from food can be a means of confirming spiritual intentions and reminding oneself that, contrary to survival instincts, a higher power sustains life, not food alone.

I met a yogi known as the Milk Baba. He was a skinny old man with long dreadlocks piled high on his head, a walking stick, and the orange robes of a Sanyasi, or spiritual renunciate. He came from a long line of yogis who, as part of their devotion to yoga, would vow not to participate in certain activities that hold an empty promise of fulfillment. The Milk Baba gave up food. For thirty-two years, he had nothing but a little milk each day. He didn't even drink water. Despite his ascetic diet, his eyes were bright and wise, he smiled a lot, and though thin, he was healthy and strong. When I met him, I asked the Milk Baba how he was feeling, having only consumed milk for thirty years. "Fine," he told me, "no problems, very happy." He told me that about seven years before he had started getting very bad migraine headaches, so he went to a doctor in India. The doctor gave him pills for the headaches, so now he still drinks only milk while taking his migraine pills. I don't recommend his diet to anyone, but I must admit he was one of the shiniest, happiest people I've ever seen.

My encounter with the Milk Baba reminded me that it's not necessarily food that keeps the body alive, even though that may seem to be the case. There is a larger force at work supporting our existence. Therese Neumann, a contemporary and friend of the well-known yogi Paramahansa Yogananda, is another example of someone who lived without food. A Christian mystic and saint, she was world famous for being a breatharian, or living only on air. There were those who doubted that such a miracle could really be happening. She agreed to let a team of scientists examine her feces for a period of six months, and no traces of food were found.

Fasting pops up in almost every religious and spiritual scripture out there. Almost every time prayer is mentioned in the Bible, it is accompanied by fasting. In ancient Judaism, fasting was a means to attain altered states of consciousness, and it is still a part of Jewish tradition. Jesus fasted for forty days and forty nights before he started teaching. Fasting has always been a way of proclaiming to the universe that you are serious about your intentions—you mean business. Even if fasting is done only for the physical benefits, an intense spiritual deepening just might happen anyway.

Yogis say that physical restraint is a basic prerequisite to power. If you fast with strong spiritual intentions to grow, improve, and change, you are empowering yourself and your ability to focus your mind. You become armed with positivity.

Fasting can also make you more sensitive to your intuition. The body and soul are able to tune in to each other, nourishing each other, focusing on a common purpose, and tuning in to the infinite. Many people experience clarity around issues that were foggy and confusing before the cleansing. Food offers gratification of the senses, but to exercise restraint by denying these senses their commonplace satisfaction elevates them to higher levels of awareness.

A typical reaction to the idea of fasting is the fear of starvation and death. I must emphasize that it is crucial to fast under the supervision of a health care professional. You must find the fast that is right for your personal physical and spiritual needs. You can do a juice fast, a fruit fast, a broth fast, a water fast, or even a monofast—during which you eat one type of fruit for a few days. Through lengthy—and supervised—water fasts, people have cured themselves of serious, supposedly fatal, diseases. It's important to determine how toxic you are and how rapidly you can handle detoxing. If you are extremely toxic and detox too quickly, you may experience detox symptoms like headache, nausea, and skin rashes. Be conscious of what you're doing, and trust someone knowledgeable to supervise your cleansing process. And no matter what, drink lots of pure water to help flush your system.

Fasting can change your body by physiologically resetting your patterns of assimilation. It can also change your relationship with the food you eat, breaking addictive behavior and deepening your understanding of what sustains your life. For those who have never fasted before, it's common to scream and run away from whoever dares to suggest you give up your daily feedings for one, three, seven, or even ten days. But for those who have been around this block, the truth is that fasting can be very beneficial to your health.

Pesticides, food additives, heavy metals in air pollution (like lead), anesthetics, residue from pharmaceutical drugs, alcohol, tobacco, and caffeine build up in your body's tissues. If you exist in this modern world, you're undoubtedly a walking sack of toxic soup. Most drinking water contains more than seven hundred chemicals (they don't boil away when you cook with tap water), and more than three thousand chemicals can be legally added to food without being listed as ingredients anywhere on the packaging. Heavy metals are especially hard on the body, often lodging in tissues and organs as a last resort after the body fails to eliminate them naturally. A toxic body can put you in a permanent bad mood, cause autoimmune disorders like fibromyalgia or cancer, and make you smell really bad.

When you fast, your digestive process shuts down after about a day—sometimes sooner. The energy that would normally be directed toward digesting food and then dealing with assimilating and eliminating is redirected toward purifying your body. Every animal in the world intuitively stops eating when it's sick for the same reason yogis fast: It gives your body the signal to clean house and let go of any crap (sometimes literally) that it didn't have time to deal with while it was busy trying to figure out what to do with the Big Mac you inhaled. Your body knows what to do when you fast—it's genetically a very natural thing to do. The body flushes out toxins that may have been accumulating for years.

11. LOVE YOUR FOOD, APPRECIATE YOUR FOOD—IT'S ABOUT TO BECOME YOU

If a person eats with anger, the food turns to poison.
—Sufi saying

A yogi wants to be conscious and alert throughout every act of life. Food is a prime means to becoming unconscious, along the same lines as TV, drugs, and other numbing vices. So from a yogic point of view, whether you're fat or thin is not an issue; it's whether you're alert and conscious of what you're doing to the body that is of the utmost significance. A true yogi is full of love, and this love extends to the body. A yogi gives conscious love and appreciation to the body and would never knowingly do anything to hurt it.

Most people don't eat out of true hunger or the intention to care for the body. Usually, there's some emotion driving it. There's some *lack* that's trying to be fulfilled through food—a compulsion being acted out through consumption. As a person who's eaten what many would call a rabbit food diet for many years, I've gone out to dinner with friends only to eat a bowl of strawberries while everyone else chows down on enormous meals. I can attest to the fact that people essentially get into a feeding frenzy—like sharks. Their eyes glaze over as they stuff themselves. It's mesmerizing to watch. Trying to fill a spiritual void with something like food just doesn't work. Why eat yourself numb? What is it you're avoiding? You can eat and eat and eat, but what are you really hungry for?

If you know why you are the shape, size, and physical condition that you are, and you desperately want to change it but somehow you just can't control yourself, ask yourself, who is this "you" that can't control "yourself"? Your relationship to yourself will be reflected in every experience you have, eating or otherwise. It's important to make this relationship a harmonious one, and to eat in a loving way.

You May Call These Foods "Comfort Foods"

People eat for many, many reasons, but not many people eat for the health of the body. Most people choose what they eat for social reasons, usually to fit in, to go out to eat with friends, or else they've been brainwashed by huge food corporations and television commercials to believe their supermarket choices are wise. Or they're simply eating the way their parents ate: "French fries were good enough for Mama, so they're good enough for me!"

I can hear you crying, "Wait! No! Don't take away my comfort food!" Well, maybe now is the time to begin seeking comfort somewhere other than in your food—especially if you're worried about being fat, or, much worse, unconscious. Seeking comfort in food is just a habit, and a habit is just a repetitive thought acted out compulsively. So change the thought. Look at it. See it for what it is, stop sleepwalking, and start acting consciously. This is the beginning of waking up.

There is such a thing as food addiction. It's so common, most people who are addicted to food believe their eating habits are normal. But watch what happens when you ask someone to give up chocolate for one week—or sugar or potatoes—just to see if they can. When going through withdrawal, this person is likely to become irritable, have physical symptoms including headaches and nausea, and display a host of other typical withdrawal symptoms (begging for just a little taste). Breaking a food addiction is just like breaking any other addiction. It requires self-examination. It requires self-forgiveness. It requires letting go of the belief that food is going to satisfy you or complete you.

You can also become addicted to self-destructive tendencies. And in terms of food, that can mean becoming addicted to food you know is bad for you simply for the knowledge of self-injury. It's a kind of escape, painting over deeper issues with smaller, more obvious ones (junk food and health problems). Unacknowledged, repressed, unexpressed emotions can be buried by addiction, only to thrive and fester in the dark. But your issues can only truly be dissolved by acknowledging them and letting them go (not by swallowing them).

Love Your Food

On one of my many trips to India, I was bitten by a mosquito carrying dengue fever. I've never been as sick as I was from that brief encounter. For days, I lay in bed in more pain than I ever imagined possible. There were moments of agony so excruciating that I would close my eyes for what seemed like hours and hours of sweaty pain, only to open them and discover that the clock claimed barely a minute had passed. It was torture, but I was lucky enough to be cared for by some good friends.

I was also lucky enough to be treated by a brilliant Ayurvedic herbalist my friend had summoned to help me. Immediately after taking some of his herbs the pain subsided enough for me to sit up in bed. The herbalist asked me why I had refused the milk offered to me by his assistant. I explained to him my belief that milk is better for calves than for me. He smiled and asked me, "What is your favorite food when you are at home?" I told him, "Salad." He said, in a thick Indian accent, "But that milk *is* a salad." At that moment, I thought he was crazy and regretted taking his herbs. He continued, "You see, lettuce and other vegetables grow from the earth, do they not? And little rabbits and other animals eat those vegetables, and those vegetables are transformed into rabbits and other animals, are they not? And those little animals do not live very long: They are eaten by tigers and transformed into tigers, are they not? And those tigers die of old age. And those tigers rot and are transformed into the earth, are they not? And that earth transforms itself into grass, does it not? And who eats that grass? Cows. And cows transform that grass into milk, do they not? So you see, the milk is a delicious salad that has been through many exciting transformations. And if you drink that milk that was once salad, it will be transformed into *you*.

"There are no vegetables." He clapped his hands emphatically. "There are no animals." He clapped again. "There is only consciousness passing through many forms." He laughed at the cleverness of his story. I told him I did see his point, but I still didn't want any milk. He told me he didn't drink milk either, that he was just making a point. Then he clapped his hands and laughed again.

From one point of view, every bit of this universe is as much your body as you are. We are inextricably intertwined with everything! From another point of view, there does seem to be some intelligence in the universe. Just like combining the colors yellow and blue will consistently make green, the combination of certain foods and your body will consistently produce certain health effects.

Even so, it's important to be aware of the essential truth: In its essence, all food is just another form of God. Your food is you and you are your food. If you think you are separate, you are mistaken. When you eat something, you are not just pushing it in one end of a tube and then pushing it out through the other end later. When you eat, your food is transformed into you—it physically becomes you. Like making love, it is a union, a yoga. It's especially important to feel gratitude for what you eat, to love what you eat, to bless what you eat.

The body is constantly sloughing off old, dead cells and replacing them with new ones. In fact, you get a completely new set of bone cells every three months, a new sack of skin every three days, a new stomach lining every four days, a new set of eye cells every two days, and a new liver every six weeks. And the food that you eat is transformed into the cells that make up your body. If you send negative energy or, worse, indifferent energy into the food you eat, that energy becomes part of you.

In a study in Japan conducted by Masaru Emoto, M.D., and Dr. Lee H. Lorenzen, a biochemist and water researcher, different words were written on bottles of water, and then the water was photographed at the cellular level with a magnetic resonance analyzer. The water that had the words *love* and *thanks* written on its bottles was beautiful, literally glowing, and perfectly symmetrical, like a snowflake. The water cells from the bottles with words like *get lost* and *die* looked brownish, partially collapsed, asymmetrical, and chaotic. The implications of this study are huge. Science is only just beginning to prove what yogis have always known to be true.

Electromagnetic energy, one of the four known forces of energy in the universe, is everywhere, in everything. Like atomic glue, it's what prevents the atoms, electrons, and neutrons that make up our cells from flying to the corners of the universe. And electromagnetic energy vibrates at many different frequencies. We're floating in a sea of frequencies, each one constantly affecting another.

12. PRACTICE YOGA

Refined over thousands of years of practice by devoted yogis, this perfect exercise harmonizes and integrates spiritual, mental, and physical energies, revealing your natural state of perfect health and unending happiness. Yogis can develop the ability to speed up or slow down their pulse at will. They've been studied by scientists and doctors because many exhibit control over functions long thought to be out of conscious control, like the actions of the thyroid and the stomach. You don't have to practice yoga every minute of every waking hour to develop and refine the functions of the body. Without ever having practiced yoga, Houdini could control muscles in the esophagus (thought to be out of the jurisdiction of conscious awareness) in order to cough up a swallowed key and release himself from the powerful chains keeping him a prisoner in a tank of water. It's a great move, but the key comes up all slimy and gooey, which is a little gross.

Yoga stimulates not only the skeletal, respiratory, and circulatory systems of the body, but more importantly, the glandular system, which controls many of the body's functions. Just by stimulating and balancing the glands, the practice of yoga postures can make you feel so rejuvenated and happy you won't feel like you need to be consoled by burying yourself in tons of food or padding yourself with fat. When you are naturally elated, you don't feel like polluting your body. You feel like loving the body—and loving everything for that matter! When you feel good, food settles into its natural place.

In my yoga class in Los Angeles, I have witnessed large, awkward bodies transform into sleek, toned, flexible, joyous yogi bodies over a period of weeks. I've even seen significant changes over a period of a few days.

Ideally, yoga postures should be practiced every day. And, as with everything, what you put into it is what you get out. If you practice for a couple of hours every day, your body will be toned, clean, and healthy. But three times a week will do wonders, too. Five minutes a day will also give you benefits. Basically, you should do your best. Do what you can and do what feels right to you; it all depends on how far you want to go with your practice, and only you can make this decision.

If I could give you only one tip about your physical yoga practice, it would be this: Try to make it fun. Enjoy your life! It's true that practicing yoga tones and cleanses all of the organs, detoxifies the body, increases circulation, oxygenates the body, balances the hormones, and prevents physical injuries, but that's only the beginning. Joy must be in the equation somewhere, otherwise it's not really yoga.

There exist some schools of yoga that teach only postures. They focus on the physical to the point of diminishing returns. Yoga is not about perfecting alignment until you look flawless. True yoga is not focused solely on externals. If you take a look at photographs of Krishnamacharya, the Indian yogi who taught the two most influential hatha yoga teachers in the world, his "alignment" is horrible, but he's clearly having a good time. He's radiant and smiling. There is a light coming from within—and that is the real yoga! It's not the direction the pinky toe is facing. Of Krishnamacharya's two influential students, one has admitted to making up all of the stringent rules and alignment theories that are currently enforced in U.S. yoga studios with the vehemence of military drills. Little did Krishnamacharya's student know what a nitpicky yoga culture he was creating! I see more sullen, miserable, sourpuss faces teaching at yoga studios than on L.A. meter maids (and they're not a happy bunch). Yoga is about joy, not preparing for military assault or joining the IRS. Don't conceal the joy, reveal it!

No one needs to hear about proper alignment more than a few times. It's like being forced to learn the alphabet every day of every year for the rest of your life, but never having the opportunity to form a word, have a conversation, or express a feeling. Physical yoga is only the beginning.

Yoga postures as they're practiced in the West are only one tiny limb of a whole system. Practicing *only* yoga postures is like driving a car with one wheel and expecting to get somewhere. Postures are part of a larger system that's designed to bring you unending happiness. In the West, yoga classes fanatically focus attention on the physical postures and alignment, but there's so much more to yoga.

True yoga is not quite as logical as the right and wrong of correct and incorrect alignment. There are no set rules and it's impossible to fail. Therefore, it's more difficult to teach—and perhaps this is why it's seldom taught. The deeper aspects of yoga must be experienced by the student directly, and this process requires more of a guide than a teacher.

By looking into yourself with the help of a good guide, you can develop a deeper understanding of your body and its role in your larger experience of life and the pursuit of its truth. Did you know that elephants can smell rain that's more than fourteen miles away? But this skill is not something they're born with; it's learned. Elephants pass down this technique from generation to generation in a beautiful ritual. All of the elephants get in a circle, with the young ones closely huddled in. All at once, the adult elephants throw their trunks up, point at the sky, and inhale. They leave their trunks up until the little ones put their trunks up too. And eventually, the little ones learn to associate that beautiful smell with the coming of the rain, like their elders. Once they can smell it, they're able to sense it for the rest of their lives. This is similar to how the true yoga has been handed down from teacher to student for thousands of years. Only *you* can intuit a deep sense of how to care for your body—and that includes your physical yoga practice. You must be able to sense when your body needs a rest and when to push it harder. You'll be able to sense which postures will benefit the body during any given practice. A yoga teacher passes on this practice primarily by example and can only point out the way. The rest is up to the student.

The twelve points I've just shared with you are meant to be helpful in your quest for truth, not a means to obsess over the body and your care of it. The point is to move beyond worrying about the body and to stop getting hung up on physical pain or distracted by deteriorating health. The yogic way is to perfect the body with beneficial physical habits and maintenance. The perfect body can be a great companion as you pursue deeper understanding and realization of your true, most essential nature.

TIPS FOR PERFECTING THE BODY

❊ Stop functioning on your programming. Think for yourself and feel for yourself. There's a big business that profits from your insecurities; don't let the corporations think for you. You know what's best for your body. Do it.

❊ Stay close to the source. Your body will do better on food that comes directly from the earth than foods made and stored in labs. The closer to its natural state, the more nourishment food has for the body.

❊ Raw reminder. When animals were fed a cooked diet they developed human diseases: arthritis, cancer, and so on. That's a clue.

❋ Don't get milk. Cow's milk is designed for calves, contains residual antibiotics, steroids, and hormones, and has been denatured by the pasteurization process. Have you been brainwashed by the movie stars in magazines with milk moustaches? Don't believe the hype.

❋ Meat ain't what it used to be. Bad feed, unnatural lifestyles and slaughter, antibiotics, hormones, steroids, acidity, and bad vibrations—need I say more?

❋ Alkalize. Acidity is a breeding ground for disease.

❋ Don't overstuff. Calorie restriction (low calorie/high nutrients) is the only known way to extend the life span and enhance health of all species.

❋ Try a fast. Fasting breaks addictive behavior and deepens your understanding of what sustains your life.

❋ Drink more water. Water can't be replaced by tea, juice, colas, and so on. Drink reverse osmosis or home-distilled water every day—an extreme minimum of ½ gallon a day up to a gallon (or more, depending on your activity level).

❋ High protein isn't the answer. Too much protein leeches calcium out of bones, causing osteoporosis. Look at the people who recommend high protein diets—they age very badly. There's a reason!

❋ Eat EFAs (essential fatty acids). Two tablespoons of flaxseed oil a day is truly all the fat the body needs (and wants). More than that is just feeding the undertaker.

❋ Exercise is important. Yoga postures are a supreme form of exercise because they aid microcirculation all over the body. I've seen some Indian yogis, even on the horrific Indian diet, who look sixty even at one hundred.

❋ State of mind is important. A victim mentality can sabotage even an otherwise very healthy lifestyle. Relax, be happy, and recognize the perfection of what is.

✳ You are not your body. You're 99.9 percent empty space and a little bit of vibrating energy. So don't be limited by what you perceive in the mirror. Look at yourself from a higher point of view, and don't worry.

SUPPLEMENTS THAT HELP

A good multivitamin will help you endlessly. Take one every day. It's very important to find a high-quality supplement that can be easily assimilated by the body.

Enzymes in the form of a supplement help your body assimilate everything you eat. Enzymes also support the pancreas, allowing it to create metabolic enzymes that repair, transform, and renew the body.

Conjugated linoleic acid (CLA) helps reduce body fat while maintaining lean muscle mass. If you're on the quest to get lean, this may help considerably. On top of everything else, it also seems to reduce the risk of cancer.

YOGA POSTURES FOR A SLEEK FORM

Surya Namaskar (Sun Salutation)

This whole series of movements is called a vinyasa, or flow. The series here is just one variation of the sun salutation. You can repeat this series of connected movements as many times as you want. It's great as a warm-up. The sun salutation tones, streamlines, and strengthens, and can help you work up quite a sweat. If you do enough of them, it's a serious fat burner. Try 10, then 20, until you work your way up to 100.

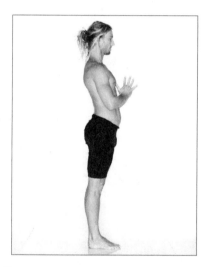

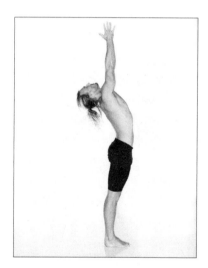

1. Begin standing, with your feet together and your hands in prayer over your heart.

2. Inhale and bring your arms over your head, tilting your head back.

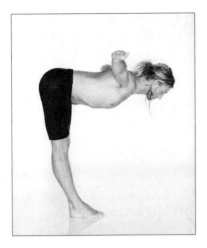

3. Exhale and swan dive into a standing forward bend . . .

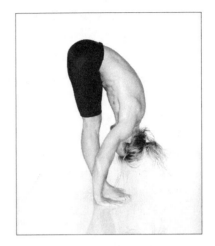

4. Place your hands at either side of your feet flat down on the mat. If your hands don't reach the mat, bend your knees.

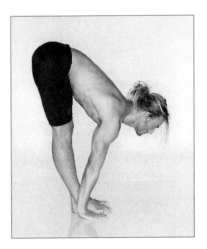

5. Lift your head and pull your chest away from your knees, flattening your back, and inhale.

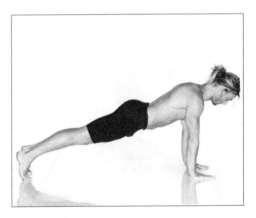

6. Exhale as you step or jump back into the top of a push-up position.

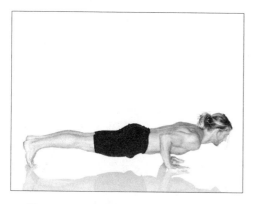

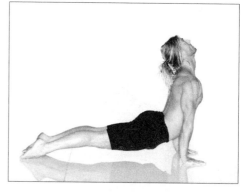

7. Keeping your elbows close to your ribs, slowly sink down to the floor, hovering a few inches off the floor.

8. From there, inhale as you push up into upward facing dog. Stay on the tops of your feet, legs straight, knees off the mat, hips off the floor, chest forward, shoulders down and back, head back, hands flat.

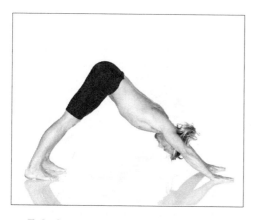

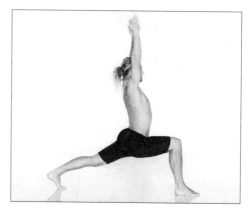

9. Exhale as you push into downward facing dog, tucking your toes under, walking your feet in slightly, and sinking your heels down. The legs are straight, the back is flat. The neck is relaxed, the chest sinks down.

10. Inhale as you bring your right foot between your hands, flat on the mat. Stay on the ball of your left foot as you bring your upper torso straight up, and lift your arms up in the air. Hold this crescent pose for 5 to 10 breaths.

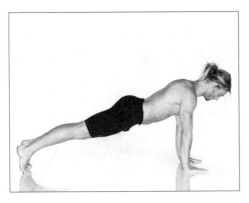

11. Inhale and bring your hands to either side of your front foot flat on the mat. Step your right foot back to the left foot and back into the top of the push-up.

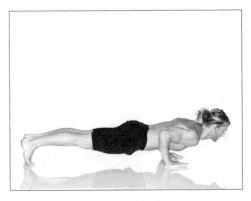

12. Exhale as you lower yourself down a couple of inches from the floor, keeping your elbows close to your body.

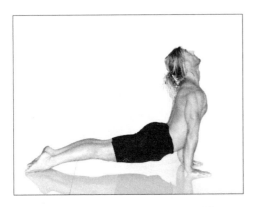

13. Inhale as you push yourself into upward facing dog. Stay on the tops of your feet, legs straight, knees off the mat, hips off the floor, chest forward, shoulders down and back, head back, hands flat.

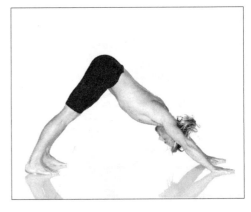

14. Exhale as you push into downward facing dog, tuck your toes under, walk your feet in slightly, and sink your heels down. The legs are straight, the back is flat. The neck is relaxed, the chest sinks down.

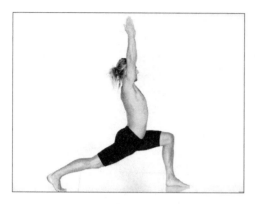

15. Inhale as you bring your left foot between your hands, flat on the mat. Stay on the ball of your right foot as you bring your upper torso straight up, and lift your arms up in the air. Hold this pose for 5 to 10 breaths.

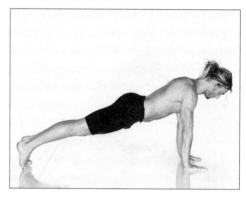

16. Inhale and bring your hands to either side of your front foot flat on the mat. Step your left foot back to the right foot and into the top of a push-up, or plank pose.

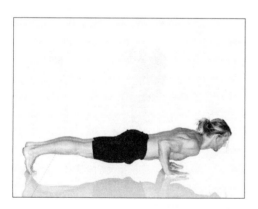

17. Exhale as you lower yourself down a couple of inches from the floor, keeping your elbows close to your body.

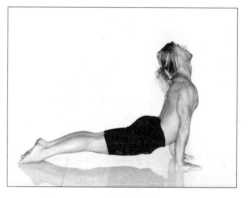

18. Inhale as you push yourself into upward facing dog. Stay on the tops of your feet, the legs are straight, the knees are off the mat, the hips are off the floor, the chest is forward, the shoulders are down and back, the head is back, the hands are flat.

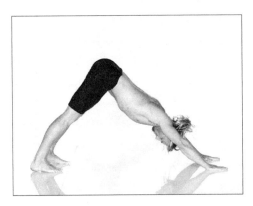

19. Exhale as you push into downward facing dog, tucking your toes under, walking your feet in slightly, sinking your heels down. The legs are straight, the back is flat. The neck is relaxed, chest sinks down.

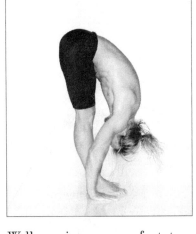

20. Walk or jump your feet to your hands, to a standing forward bend.

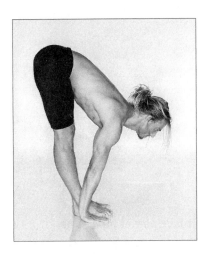

21. With your hands flat on the mat, lift your head and pull your chest away from your knees, flattening your back as you inhale.

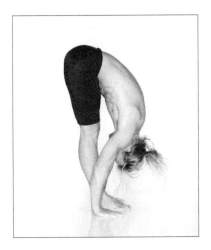

22. Exhale as you fold back into a standing forward bend.

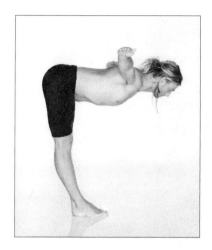

23. Inhale and bring your arms up to the sides . . .

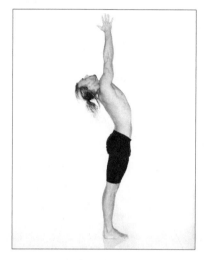

24. . . . and then over your head. Hold them straight and tilt your head back.

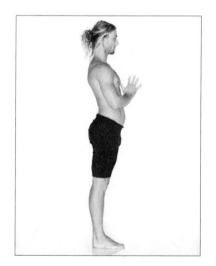

25. Exhale as you bring your hands to prayer position over your heart.

Repeat as many times as you want.

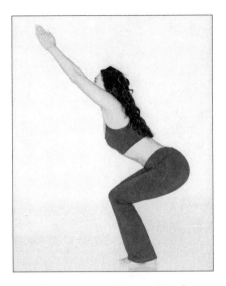

UTKATASANA (CHAIR POSE)

Stand with your feet and knees together. Bend your knees to a 45-degree angle, put your weight on your heels, and bring your arms straight up above you. To intensify the pose, press your palms together above your head. Look up and keep the chest lifted. Really squeeze the legs together, engage the abdominals, and stretch the upper body toward the ceiling. Breathe. Hold the pose for 30 seconds to 1 minute.

When done properly, this pose tones the body from head to toe, streamlining and strengthening.

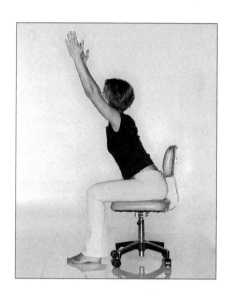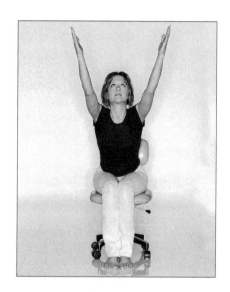

UTKATASANA—AT DESK VARIATION

Sitting in a chair with your legs and ankles together, squeeze your legs into each other like you're holding a pencil between your thighs.

Bring your arms over your head, look up, lift the chest, engage the abdominals, and tuck the butt slightly under. Hold for 45 seconds or more.

PLAYLIST SUGGESTIONS

1. "Get Jiggy Wit' It" · Will Smith
2. "Mustang Sally" · The Commitments
3. "Signed, Sealed, and Delivered" · Stevie Wonder
4. "Gonna Make You Sweat" · Inner Circle
5. "I Am a Queen" · India Arie
6. "Gettin' Hot in Here" · Nelly
7. "Isn't She Lovely" · Stevie Wonder

⇴ REASON 4 ⇴

YOU ARE NOT YOUR DAILY GRIND
(PRECISELY WHO DO YOU THINK YOU ARE?)

If you're driven to be successful in life, you are truly blessed. Without the urge to be better, to reach goals, and to strive, complacency can set in, halting the natural growth of any being. But what is it that you're seeking from your career? Do you believe that your daily grind is going to take you to a higher level of awareness, or just to a bigger house with a view? As a yogi, you must keep in mind that once you've moved into your mansion, it's still you who has moved in. And who are you?

For a long time, India was one of the most affluent places on the planet. Singular in its trade of spices, silk, gold, and jewels, India was a land of kings. Many of the wealthy landowners, monarchs, and traders fulfilled every single one of their worldly desires. They wanted land? They got it. They wanted power? They got it. They wanted feasts? No problem. They wanted the latest technology? Done. What does the person who has everything, can buy anything, and has all of the power do next? If you have everything you have ever desired, yet still feel emptiness—a yearning for fulfillment—what do you do? Many of these overachieving Indians chose to become disciples of great sages and enlightened teachers. And many of them attained enlightenment. They knew worldly, materialistic acquisitions wouldn't satisfy them. They'd tried. Certain the phenomenal world was full of empty promises, they became fervent, sincere seekers of the truth while maintaining their wealth, power, and kingdoms.

At the moment, we are not so dissimilar to the Indian kings of the past. Like them, we have the potential to meet every desire—almost instantly. Never before have humans had such decadent luxuries. Even what we consider the simplest conveniences—heated running water, the ability to be anywhere in the world in a matter of hours, fast "food," twenty-four-hour televised entertainment—would seem lavish and extravagant indulgences to humans in less privileged societies and eras. Instant gratification is practically everywhere. Even many of our homeless and jobless are satisfied to the point of being a little chubby in the belly. Throughout history, all over the world, a little fat on the belly has been a privilege enjoyed exclusively by the rich. Our poorest in the West are an earlier century's fortunate in terms of physical luxuries.

We are the kings of the consumer world. If we can dream it up, industry can produce it and sell it to us. Even if we can't dream it up, industry can sell it to us. Here we are, kings of our domain.

We're lucky to have the opportunity to experience life in a time and place in which every daydream of future fulfillment can be realistically achieved in a relatively short period of time. Setting goals and achieving every one of them can be a great practice. Once you have money, power, lovers, fame, respect, and lots of cool stuff, perhaps only then will you be brave enough to encounter the final frontier of the soul. If you've got everything the world can give you, if you're living in a house with diamond walls, you have ten cars and six motorcycles, and still it's not enough, still you're unsatisfied, then perhaps as you gaze out at the ocean from your own private island in the Caribbean, you'll feel a subtle certainty flow through every inch of your being, a certainty that what's outside of you is never going to fulfill you completely. There's something more to this life, and it's found by turning within.

Having things and experiences are fine, but they will never bring you lasting peace and happiness. Wake up!

⚔ THE HUNGRY GHOST REALM ⚖

You do not need to leave your room. Remain sitting at your table and listen. Do not even listen, simply wait. Do not even wait, be quite still and solitary. The world will freely offer itself to you unmasked, it has no choice, it will roll in ecstasy at your feet.
—Franz Kafka

If you were a king in India, the first thing your spiritual teacher would warn you about is the most common pitfall of all pitfalls, the easiest to slip into, and the most difficult to drag yourself out of: the hungry ghost realm. This is a term used by both yogis and Buddhists to describe a place—or a state of mind—where beings wander and dart, never seeing one another, never taking anything in, never enjoying the moment, always mulling over the future or the past, and always feeling very alone, despite being surrounded by other hungry ghosts exactly like themselves. Hungry ghosts are possessed by desire. If they see something they think they can't have, they immediately become consumed by their lust for it. It is not a realm of having. As soon as something is acquired, it's immediately ignored and wasted. A hungry ghost wouldn't even be aware of having, because once a thing is had, a new want arises and consumes every nook and cranny of the now even hungrier ghost's being. There's no room for having when you're full of wants. Hungry ghosts are constantly wondering, "What's next?"

A hungry ghost's mind and identity has become consumed by a long list of desires. There's always something more to jones after. A hungry ghost would be the last being to see itself as a hungry ghost, because it still believes strongly in the appearances of the phenomenal world—a world that seems to be full of promises. The promises, however, always fail to deliver satisfaction. Like a drug addict or a compulsive gambler, the hungry ghost is oblivious to this seemingly obvious pattern. Nothing is ever good enough once they *get* it, and everything is perfect when it's just out of reach. *The hungry ghost's main attribute is absolutely insatiable desire*—constant and relentless wanting and craving.

These characteristics might be a little familiar to you, either in people you've encountered or even in yourself. You want a new motorcycle, and you get it (or not), and then you want a racer boat, and you get it (or not), and then you want new carpeting, and you get it (or not), and then you want a new television, and you get it (or not), and every time you get something (or not), you feel satisfied for a split second, and then you feel emptier than before. Some people wake up to this cycle and some people don't.

If you don't catch on to the pattern, eventually even you can become a vacuous, bottomless pit of wants. Your life becomes about trying to get stuff, often complaining about what you don't have (either out loud or in your thoughts), with very little of anything else left (especially integrity, love, or peace of mind). The hungry ghosts don't see themselves that way, of course, and to try to point it out is a doomed endeavor. There's no room left in that type of awareness for anything other than desires, and the ego-mind justifies it any way it can. Be careful not to get caught in this emptiness—it's a long, dark journey to nowhere.

Hungry ghosts typically get caught in a downward spiral of want, lack, and poverty. This is a major problem if you're a yogi aspiring toward a higher, more profound experience of life. Energy, attention, and awareness—the keystones of a yoga practice—are consumed with wanting, leaving you stuck wrestling with the everyday superficialities of life. *Having*, on the other hand, requires much less attention and energy. Once you are no longer desperately seeking satisfaction, but feeling satisfied, the world will do everything it can to further satisfy you. It delivers itself to you on a platter. Having can take you to a place of maturity where you can deal with deeper questions of existence and attain enlightenment.

⚜ ARE YOU THE DREAM OR THE DREAMER? ⚜

Understand that the Self is eternal and always Here!
—H.W.L. Poonjaji

⟶═◉═⟵

When you're asleep and dreaming, if a snake bites you, you feel it in the dream. You scream in the dream, you bleed in the dream, you writhe around in pain in the dream. While you're dreaming, that snakebite is your real, genuine experience. But when you wake up, the wound, the pain, and the teeth marks are gone because in fact they were never there. Even though it was just a dream, that doesn't mean the bleeding, the wound, and the pain weren't your true experience while you were dreaming. It was. But then you wake up and you know that you're safe in your bed. And that is also your true, genuine experience.

The yogis also like to reflect on the vicious tiger that hunts you in your dream. You're running, you're panting, you're sweating, and then you wake up. Where did that tiger go? You're now cozy in your bed, but where is that tiger? It was just a kind of hallucination, but as it was happening, it seemed unquestionably real. But from the waking perspective, who you thought you were in that dream, who you thought you should be, what you thought was happening disappears. From one perspective, the tiger in your dream was absolutely real. You could see it, hear it, feel it—it was real! From another perspective, it was an absolute illusion. Once you wake up, you can remember some of the details of your experience, and yet you're unharmed, safe, and secure in your comfortable bed. From that point of view, it was not real. From the waking state, you might even feel silly for becoming so upset while you were dreaming. But while you're dreaming, you're usually unaware that it's just a dream. So, was that tiger real? And the venom you saw oozing from the snake's teeth and into your flesh—was that real? The ultimate truth contains both aspects of duality: The hunting tiger and the poisonous snake are both real and not real at the same time, depending on your perspective.

This same dynamic can be applied to the experience of living. In this life, your daily existence seems urgent, often stressful. It probably seems that your day-to-day life is all there is to your being. That's true from one point of view—the yogis would call it the dreaming point of view. From the point of view of the awakened soul, there's a bit more to it than that. Yes, life is happening. But at the same time, you become aware of the soul's journey. You become aware that like all dreams, this one will end. And you become aware of your essence, the part of you that was aware before this life began and will continue to be aware after this life ends. Once you wake up to this dream, who are you then? Who is the dreamer?

Dreams come and go, and so do lives, identities, bodies, roles, jobs, situations, lovers, snakes, and tigers. One thing remains the same as the dreams change: the dreamer. So the real question becomes, who is dreaming? This is far more important than the drama of the dream.

From the point of view of the yogi, life is precious only in its potential to reveal who you really are. Names, places, and possessions are not ends in and of themselves. Rather, they are the means to discover who is aware of them. It rains? Fine. Who is aware of this rain? You got promoted? Great. Who is aware of this promotion? I think you get the picture: Your life situation is not something that must be solved and perfected, but something that—regardless of its positive or negative appearance—gives you the opportunity to realize the deepest truth of your existence.

There is a degree of freedom in the very nature of this quest. The drama of the world loses its grip on you when you stop believing the characters and situations are permanent or truly threatening. When you realize the dreamer—your awareness—is the only one that warrants examination, the dream—this life—becomes much more fun. The snake becomes a friendly character, fascinating instead of terrifying; the tiger is your friend, pointing you toward realization. Instead of screaming, you might thank him for such an exciting, challenging chase through the jungle.

The events of this life—"I have to do this, do that, get there, meet him, *or else*"—become less of a constant emergency. The urgency dissolves, and you calmly go from encounter to encounter, enjoying every moment to its fullest, without fear. The world tends to bend toward a fearless being; life becomes peaceful, fluid, easy, and beautiful. In this way, enlightenment is a very practical state. If you could have a perfect, wonderful, joyous experience of life, wouldn't you?

Can you dream and be awake at the same time? Yes. You can be present in your life story and also aware of that part of you that has no beginning and no end. It's simply a matter of expanding your awareness. All that separates any person from the ultimate awareness of this life are the obfuscations of the mind. In truth you are perfectly safe, happy, and peaceful no matter what seems to happen around you. How buried that awareness of the ultimate truth is in the muck and mire of dreams, fantasies, memories, and compulsive thinking varies. But this much is always true: You can find your true, limitless Self.

It's one thing to understand all of this intellectually; it's a very beautiful concept. But how can you integrate it into your experience? The walls around your true self must be penetrated, the many layers of the onion have to be peeled away, to reach that beautiful, perfect center of pure peace and energy. This process of undoing is the heart of yoga. There have been many methods, workshops, and fad New Age books addressing this quest for peace, but all roads don't lead to Rome. There are lots and lots of really slow boats that are largely for wallowing and indulging the intellectual mind. Taking one of these detours can leave you settled down in a small village near the suburbs of Rome, or even in the outskirts of the small village near the suburbs. It's good to be *almost* at peace with yourself, to almost know, but you don't have to settle for almost.

Over countless thousands of years, yoga has developed a track record for turning out fully enlightened beings. Like the Buddha, most fully realized beings have been yogis emerging from the yoga motherland, India. The yogis know a few things that can get you to the heart of Rome by jet plane, but you don't have to go to India to integrate yogic teachings into your life. You can be driven for success, on the hot rod track for triumphant commercial achievements, and also become enlightened, or at least blissfully happy. It has been done. Some truth seekers believe you can't live in this culture that revolves around ambition and apparent success—that you have to travel to Burma, India, or Tibet to be yogic. But enlightenment is not geographically located. Inner peace is possible anywhere and in any situation. It is within you! You are just as likely to reach full enlightenment in your current situation as the Buddha was in his—if you make it your *first* priority.

Once you realize who the dreamer is, you become empowered to dream any dream you choose. You become free to have any experience—rich, famous, powerful, brilliant, and even enlightened. It all becomes so easy.

Who are you? Ooo, ooo, ooo, ooo.
— **The Who**

⊰⊙⊱

If you ask the average person who they are, you'll get the usual responses: "I am a mother." "I am a CEO." "I am a security guard." "I am a grandfather." If you ask how they are, you'll get the everyday, "I am good," "I am happy," "I am sad," "I am depressed," "I am ecstatic." All of the words that follow the phrase "I am" are identifications. And on one level, they're all true, but these identifications can be extremely limiting. If you think that's *all* you are, you're tying yourself to a very limited identity—one that leads to intensified duality (i.e., suffering). If you strongly identify with being a high-powered executive, you may have great success in that field. You may also be miserable in every other area of your life. That's intensified duality.

Buying a sweater that you've seen seemingly happy people wear might lead you to believe that when you wear it, you'll be happy. That's trying to buy and wear an identity. In truth, all you get is the sweater. Expecting happiness from an identity you've purchased is delusional. The same is true when you think the role of mother, father, president, or millionaire will make you totally happy. In and of itself, an identification won't make you happy. That's not to say that being a factory worker, a father, a doctor, or a dog walker is bad. It's to say that *this is not all you are.* Essentially, identities are what differentiate you from other people, but they also reinforce the ego's conviction that you are separate from God. You're not.

Yoga seeks to discover that which has no beginning and no end. What is lasting? What is permanent? What is the essence of being? If your primary identity is that of being a mother, you may have a happy life as long as that lasts. Your clothes, home, lifestyle, friends, car, and activities may revolve around and support this identity. This identity defines you, helps you make life decisions, and delineates where you end and where someone else begins. It is your own personal boundary. You may find some fulfillment in this identity, but what happens when the children grow up, leave the house, and don't want you to hover around their comings and goings anymore? An identity crisis is what happens: If being a mother can no longer be your primary identity, what are you? Who are you now?

Deriving your identity from anything in this world and expecting it to bring you fulfillment will inevitably bring disappointment. Everything is temporary. What if you derive your identity from being a wealthy investment banker? You have plenty of money and rich friends, you shop at fancy stores, and your taste is superlative. That might be really fun until the stock market crashes. If these elements are the sole source from which you have derived your identity, you might find yourself jumping out of your office window on a fateful black Monday. Why? Because if what you suppose is your identity is annihilated, your sense of who you are, of where you collect fulfillment, of why you think you receive love, and of where you fit in are all eradicated. Some people try to move from one identity to another as a form of survival. When the identity of an investment banker stops working, you might transition to being a house husband. But what happens when the children grow up? You'll have to find yet another identity. Adapting to change is necessary and may keep you from feeling suicidal, but in the end, every identity expires and has limitations.

On a practical level, you can define yourself, organize your life, set goals, achieve them, and do all the things that are typically deemed healthy and productive. However, ultimately this alone will not be totally satisfying. There's nothing wrong with functioning easily in the world. Smooth functioning will typically get you more smooth functioning and a lot of neat stuff, but it probably won't take you to enlightenment. You may even believe that if you define yourself more and more, you will someday define yourself into satisfaction. Guess again! It is more likely that you'll end up defining yourself into a cage, resulting in despair.

Have you built your life around your identifications? Have you painted yourself into a corner? Do you think you're your job? Your trophy spouse? Your musical preference? Your wardrobe? Having very rigid identifications is like overfurnishing a house. Every space becomes so cluttered and packed with stuff that you can't even travel from one room to another. Being free of false identifications is like going to a national park and standing in the middle of a wide open field: clear air, unobstructed freedom of movement, and infinite potential.

When you stop looking to your worldly identifications for fulfillment, your energy shifts and the mind has the potential to be clear and free. You can still take on the role of the mother and enjoy it completely, but you can drop it, too. You can still be an investment banker, but when that stops working you can drop it and take on the role of a painter if you want. You can also drop all identifications and just be as you are. This often takes the most courage but also holds the most power and freedom.

There's bliss in letting go of your habitual identifications. You might think you are your appearance—a pretty girl, a GQ man, a dorky guy—but when you drop that identification, you might be able to have a lot more fun with your appearance. The heaviness of the identification, the need to be fulfilled by your appearance is lifted.

This is where finding yourself comes in. To find the absolute essence of who you are, you must acknowledge the identifications you've already latched on to. Look at them closely: Do you think you're an artist, a movie star, a janitor, a genius, an assistant, a teacher, a mother, a father, a child, an adult, a good person, or a bad person? Now look past them. Look through them. Beyond all of your identifications, who are you? What is your essence? Getting to know yourself doesn't require any additional words, thoughts, or labels. It is an undoing, a feeling, a knowing. It is peace.

INNER YOGA

1. Who do you think you are? Make a list.

2. Now, just for a moment, imagine you are no longer any of those identities. What's left of you? Who is aware of what's left?

⊰ MEMORIES AND FANTASIES ⊱

Beyond identification with roles—doctor, trapeze artist, student—lurks an even more limiting one: identification with the past and the future. How deeply entrenched and vast are the stories that fill most minds with beliefs and opinions revolving around events that may happen in the future or have happened in the past? And how much mental energy is designated to these thoughts of the nonexistent past and future? Like the toys on a baby's mobile revolving above the crib, they're the same thoughts spinning round and round. To an infant, each object looks brand new when it reaches his line of vision. He's not aware enough to notice the repetition. The toy appears constantly new because it moves, just as events move in time. But it's not new, it's just the same brightly colored distraction going around in circles, entertaining the infant mind.

In a similar manner, the ego recites these past and future thoughts over and over again like an elaborate novel. The ego will continue this mental game of smoke and mirrors until your awareness develops enough to see the patterns. As you become more conscious, more aware, you will question this mental merry-go-round. Is that thought really a brand-new horse, or have you seen it two million times already this week? What is true? All that is really true is happening in this moment. The rest is just the content of the mind.

What if you are not your past or your future? What if you are not your opinions or your judgments? What if you are not your daily dramas? What then?

When meeting someone for the first time, it's pretty common to swap life stories. "Well, I grew up here, and I went to school there. My mother was this way, and my father was this way. I want to do this, I want to be this." I'm sure you've heard it all a thousand times. You might even be tired of hearing your own story. Why not drop it? The past is over with and the future is truly unknown. So what's the point of giving either of them one more second of your life? Why not enjoy this moment as it is, unfettered by limiting mind stuff and stories struggling to define and confine you? If you hear enough of them, they begin to sound like exactly what they are, stories—a series of events tied together by opinions and related characters, with tragic and/or comedic undertones. They can form an enticing stage play, but they're not really an accurate reflection of who anyone is in this moment. In any given moment, memories, histories, and past events are really only thoughts. You can't do anything with the past and the future except think about them—they only exist in the mind. Thoughts get distorted with time, colored by projections of the future (also only thoughts), and your own desires to define yourself at the expense of the truth. Thoughts of the past and the future can pull on each other, distorting and twisting your perception of the moment. Is this any way to get to know a person or even yourself? Is this really who anyone is— a grocery list of identifications and stories?

Stop thinking. Look around. What's happening? This moment is all there is.

Becoming aware of your stories about the future and the past, and realizing these stories are not ultimately who you are, that in fact they're limiting, is vastly liberating. To be free to perceive this moment with clarity, you must be free of future and past identifications (or at least aware of them). Do you have stories about yourself or your experience that you tell yourself and others over and over? What do these stories justify? What if your stories were fiction and everyone knew it, including you? What if you couldn't use them anymore to justify your identity? Then who would you be?

Have you ever had such a profound change in your point of view that when you look back at who you were ten years ago, that person seems like a stranger to who you are now? You might not even loan your car to the person you were ten years ago. Your awareness didn't die, but who you thought you were did pass away. It can happen once, twice, or several times in a lifetime. Changing careers, spouses, religions, or even your geographical location can radically alter who you think you are. Your identification can shift so severely that you no longer relate in the same way to anything at all. What do you think would happen if you dropped all of your identifications?

You can pop out of every new second fresh and clean, innocent like a baby and wise like a sage. Each new moment is an opportunity for rebirth. The number of habits and thoughts you carry with you from a previous life, hour, or minute is up to you. You can live each moment free from the past and the future if you stay very alert.

⊰ YOU SEE WHAT YOU BELIEVE ⊱

When a pickpocket meets a saint, all he sees are his pockets.
—Baba Hari Dass

Your identifications will color your experience. Who you are is so much bigger and broader than any identity or label can pretend to capture. Similarly, what and who you experience yourself to be all depends on how aware you are.

To a realized yogi, life looks absolutely perfect just as it is. Have faith and trust that the magic of cause and effect takes everyone through exactly what they need to go through, when they need to go through it. Resisting or flipping out in reaction to life doesn't help you, and in fact it can act to reinforce the patterns already in play. If you see life as unfair and cruel, it will show you that very dynamic in every situation and every person you meet. If you see life as beautiful and miraculous, the world will show you that over and over again. If you go through life compulsively thinking the same thoughts over and over again, and you find yourself acting out or being the victim of the same patterns over and over again, this is not a curse or a coincidence. Life is reflecting your identifications back to you in every way it can, hoping that you'll get the picture. If you can see yourself for what you really are, you will naturally see life for what it really is. It's simple yogic logic.

To the yogi, the phenomena and appearances of life are all manifestations of consciousness. Everywhere you turn, there you are. If you look at life in a yogic way, you can see that God is everywhere. And if you really pay attention, you might see that your life is constantly pointing you toward realizing your essence. In a way, your life becomes your guru. It gives you candy with one hand, then whacks you with a stick with the other. It might seem like torture, but if you're alert and a fairly quick learner, it can be a great teacher.

We are fortunate to be alive at this particular time in history. The more intense and dualistic the world and daily life become, the more powerful the impetus to wake up. Your life—and when I say your life, I mean everything you interact with on a daily basis: your morning juice, the newspaper, your children, your parents, your work, your coworkers, your boss, the checkout guy at the market, your spouse or lover, and your ideas—can be seen as provocation for waking up to your deeper experience: your soul, the Self, the part of you that's perfect just as it is.

You can become aware and experience that not only are you connected, but one with every other being. And not only are these beings teaching you, guiding you, pointing you in the right direction, but they are in fact aspects of you. If you disregard the mind's attempts to isolate and define you, you realize that they are as much *you* as you are. It's all pretty obvious when you really take a look at it.

Enlightenment is possible in this lifetime. It's only your limited mind that stands between you and your experience of yourself as an unlimited being. The first time you see someone tie their body into knots and wrap their legs around their ears, you might think it's implausible that you could someday be in the same position. And then, one day, after some practice of hatha yoga postures, you might find yourself doing what you previously thought impossible. The mind is very limited. Your experience doesn't have to be.

A yogic saint is someone who sees only the divine in the everyday experience of life. So if a saint is throwing garbage at you, what you experience is duality: the saint and the garbage vs. you. What the saint experiences is God throwing garbage at God, or better yet, God throwing God at God. He sees past the periphery of form. When a saint sees another person, he doesn't see another person. He sees God in a form, pretending not to be God. That's why yogic saints look at you with that twinkle in their eye that says, "Come on, I know you're God, quit playing around."

⫷ THE YOGI SANYASI ⫸

In India, there are yogis called sanyasi who renounce seeking fulfillment in the phenomenal world. They renounce any combination of alcohol, meat, sex, speaking, touching money, sitting (some sanyasis have stood on one leg for years at a time), or any other manifestation of worldly life. Regardless of their particular renunciation, they are just truth-seeking yogis. They're easy to spot because they normally wear bright orange robes. Most sanyasis are constantly on the move—they never stay in one place for more than three days. The idea is to form no attachments, thereby remaining free of their own identifications and the projected identities of those they meet on their journeys. By the time anyone gets to know a sanyasi, starts to form opinions, and categorize him into a neat little box, the sanyasi's on the way out of town. Not only do they not limit themselves, but they don't allow the world to limit them either. This is an extreme version of refusing identifications and the personal attachments that go with them, and yet the sanyasis seem pretty happy when you run into them. Talk about not being tied down.

To effectively practice yoga, it's not necessary to renounce material phenomena, abandon your family and friends, and go live in a log cabin in the woods. That's actually the easy way out. It's much more challenging to be in the world, surrounded by phenomena, dealing with phenomena, earning and spending phenomena, and endeavor to see through it. It might seem impressive to renounce the world, become a monk, and hide away from the severity of duality in pursuit of enlightenment. But how do you know if you have gone through all your unconsciousness if you're never challenged?

There's a yogi story about just that: A very old, wise yogi was sitting under a beautiful tree at the bank of a river. His devotee was nearby, and asked if he wanted anything. "Yes," the yogi replied, "maybe a glass of water. I'm thirsty." His devotee ran off to fetch him a glass of water. While the devotee was gone, the yogi slipped into a very deep state of samadhi. He remained in this blissful state of union with the infinite for years. Hardly breathing and his heart barely beating, he maintained a deep state of bliss. Many came to pay respect to this high being in his high state. One morning, after several years like this, the yogi's eyes popped open, and he sat up and looked around. His devotee came running to his side. "Master, master, what wisdom have you brought from the other side? Have you attained enlightenment?" The master replied, "I am very, very thirsty. Where is my glass of water?!?"

It is a deep yogic wisdom that issues and desires don't go away until they're completely, truly dissolved. The longer you keep your desires and attachments bottled up, the more they'll fester and grow. Any lingering desire will rankle and intensify until it's dealt with and released, no matter how high or pleasant a state you slip into. Preoccupying the mind is like sweeping the dirt under the carpet. The dirt may not be visible, but it's still there. So if wearing an orange robe and wandering from town to town for the rest of your life is a way of running or hiding from your desires, the life of a sanyasi will only take you further away from Self-realization. Renunciation can become just another identity, another role from which to expect satisfaction. That kind of identity can even have the element of being holier than everyone else. If that's the case, it would be just as spiritual to take on the identity of a Hollywood agent. It's just a power trip. To truly be free of your desires, you must release them. To be free of wanting is to find your source of satisfaction within.

But there is some value in the idea of worldly renunciation—and you don't have to run from the world to benefit from it. The only true renunciation is to renounce seeking fulfillment in the fluttering phenomena of the world. And you can do that anywhere, wearing any color. The world becomes even more enjoyable once you stop demanding fulfillment from it. You can play in it and you can enjoy it without expecting a single thing from it. It's beautiful, it's fun. When you stop placing expectations on your identities and the world, you begin to see that every event, every moment, is a miracle.

Once you recognize your own identifications, you can experiment with releasing them. Even if you just let go of who you think you are for five minutes, it's a good beginning. It's like taking off a sweater you've been wearing for eighty years: It's not a bad feeling to be naked for just a little while. Maybe take a shower. Rest assured you can put it back on anytime you want, but for the sake of your inner peace, try letting go of your identities and see how you feel.

INNER YOGA

1. Examine your life and your beliefs. Are you looking for fulfillment in any of your identities? (Hint: Of course you are!) If you look beyond these identifications for who you are, what do you find? What do you feel?

2. Many conflicts arise when an individual feels like his or her identity is being threatened. To defend the ego-mind's identity (as a job, a spouse, a status, a country, a sports team, a beauty, or the like), you may find yourself enmeshed in arguments or even violence. Can you remember a situation like this in your life? How about today? How about now?

⚔ YOGIS CAN MAKE MONEY ⚔

Yogis advise the relinquishment of your expectations of the world. You can also relinquish expectations of the roles you play in your life. When Russel Simmons, the founder of Def Jam Records, Phat Farm clothes, and an integral aspect of the group that created what we now know as hip hop, first started coming to my class, he just wanted some exercise while he checked out all the beautiful models and actresses sweating through their tops. You know what happens to a white shirt on a beautiful woman when she's drenched in sweat? It becomes absolutely transparent. Why do women wear white shirts to my class? I'm not sure. But it served to bring Russel back time and again. Eventually, though, the yoga took on a new and deeper meaning, and it began changing the patterns of Russel's mind. Before he knew it, he wasn't focused on the women anymore. It wasn't anything I was doing or he was doing. Inner peace was happening to him. During meditation, he felt peace as his mind slowed down and stopped for a moment. His desires subsided a little bit. He started to feel happy just as he was. Peace, joy, and stillness got into his system. One day he told me he had to stop doing yoga or he was going to lose all his money. I just laughed. To his surprise, he didn't lose his money—as a matter of fact, it was precisely at that time his fortune tripled, and it continues to grow. He still practices yoga, and inner peace is continuing to happen to him. It's a beautiful thing.

I've learned from many of my most successful students that in high-stress, high-stakes careers, you have to either learn to let go or die an early death. If you think you're controlling every outcome, manipulating each scenario, you're bound to end up in the hospital sooner or later—it's a recipe for a heart attack. Clarity and peace of mind will enhance your career. You may not feel like hustling all the time, manipulating everything and everyone every second of the day and night, but that's fine because you won't have to. One brilliant move is far more powerful than a hundred muddled, mediocre ones. Make a million dollars in one move instead of a thousand dollars in a hundred clumsy moves. Through yoga and meditation, you gain insight into everything, including your career. Situations that seem oppressively complex to the average thinker are simple to one who thinks clearly. Solutions become obvious.

Eventually, you come to realize that it doesn't matter how much success you have or don't have—you'll be fine. You'll be happy. You can keep making money if you want to—just for the fun of it—or not. For the yogi, pursuing the phenomenal world is a personal choice. For some it's fun, for others, drudgery. Some structure their lives so as to spend as much time as possible just meditating. I teach yoga classes at my studio every day and I enjoy that very much, but I find the simpler my life is, the more I am able to enjoy the satisfaction I get from being quiet and still.

You're only aware of what you focus your attention on. Life really becomes a function of what you want to experience, and therefore a result of how you focus your energy and attention. What is it you want to be aware of? If your attention is sucked into compulsive thinking, personal drama, other people's drama, business dilemmas, and so on, that's all you'll be aware of. If your attention is directed toward the truth of this existence, your awareness will be drawn deeper and deeper into that arena.

The truest sanyasi life is to renounce the ego-mind's dominance over the spirit: To watch the mind instead of believing every thought that pops out of it is the ultimate truth. It's like *watching* a con artist try to sell you a piece of real estate sight unseen instead of *believing* every word he says and giving him your life savings. It's being alert, aware, and conscious.

Watching thoughts is an extremely high yogic practice. It may not be easy at first, but when you take a look at your other options—repression, blame, or acting out—watching the ego-mind is the only sane thing to do. Repressing thoughts and emotions only makes them stronger; acting them out on other people only creates ugliness, conflict, and eventually war. And blaming the world for who and how you are reinforces a victim mentality, only adding to the cycles of negativity that are already out there. So what do you do? You undo. You yoga. Stay focused on why you're really here—to wake up.

Once a vigilant state becomes second nature, the people in the world running around, chasing their problems, following their desperation, moaning and complaining, seem to be under a collective hypnosis. It's as if the entire population has been duped into believing they are limited, powerless beings. They've been tricked—by themselves. When you wake up to the reality that love, bliss, and peace are your natural condition, all of the negativity and false identifications seem so pointless—like being fully dressed but hypnotized to believe that no matter how many layers of clothes you put on, you're still naked. You don't need to cover up your perfect, inherent beauty with identity after identity. You need nothing more than what you have. You are as complete as you ever will be. You are complete as you are.

Once the mind is quiet and thoughts stop, you can listen to the silence within you and that is where you will find every answer to every question ever asked. Regardless of your role, wealth, or wardrobe, that's the true sanyasi life.

⊰ WHAT YOUR ANALYST PROBABLY WON'T TELL YOU ⊱

Anything more than the truth would be too much.
—Robert Frost

⊷⊷◉⊷⊷

Psychoanalysis can be effective for learning how to cope with the world, and in many practical matters may be very useful. To sort out the elements of your life, organize thoughts, and make big life decisions it can be helpful to have someone reasonable and unbiased to listen objectively to you. Beyond that, however, it can turn into a festival of thinking about thoughts; trying to figure out that which cannot be figured out. The world is not a sensible place on almost any thinking level, and often analysis is a slow and very expensive process of learning how to live with and integrate nonsense. Sifting through the past, searching for answers in a world that no longer exists, and imposing meanings and judgments on the various characters in your life story is a big part of most therapy sessions. It's stimulating to the intellect and holds some consolation for those who feel wounded. But consolation is of no interest to those who are adamantly seeking the truth, breathing for the truth. Temporary consolation is an obstacle, not a goal.

It may be better than drifting through life submissively without inquiring into the mechanics of being, but therapy and analysis are limited in their scope of potential freedoms. They can only take you so far. Contemplating the grave disorder of the world and the mind won't free you of the lunacy of the human condition. You can try to understand it, but even if you get close to understanding it, that doesn't mean you will become sane yourself. It only means that you might be able to function comfortably in a madhouse. Is this truly desirable? You can presume to figure it all out, but the yogi's aim is transcendence.

I'm personally not a big fan of psychiatric medication in most cases either. In serious cases of psychosis I can see that it may be necessary, but the trend lately is to medicate every man, woman, and child until they're complacent enough—or stoned enough—to appear "normal" (whatever that is). What's wrong with experiencing an uncomfortable emotion? Nothing. Medicating a person doesn't address the problem; it only addresses a symptom. And like most modern medicine, that's like putting a Band-Aid on an erupting volcano: It's very, very temporary. Drugs are a dodge, an avoidance, stopping one problem and creating another one. The world is enough of a circus without adding that kind of cat-and-mouse entertainment. What's the root of a problem? You can't just trim back weeds; it makes them flourish. You have to get the whole problem—roots and everything—out of your system, and you probably don't have three hundred years to do it in this lifetime (unless you follow the advice in Reason 3).

The yogi's practice is to fully feel and allow an emotion, thereby going through it, as opposed to burying it or running away from it. What's at the heart of the emotion? What's underneath it? Who is it that is experiencing this emotion? These are the fundamental questions.

If you can raise your awareness of a problem to the point of view of spirit, what seemed like a giant one-eyed monster, banging around in your closet and wanting to eat you, may turn out to be just a friendly little mouse trying to get back to its field. If you can shift your point of view, or the perspective from which you witness an issue, you can see it for what it really is: just a thought. And you can see yourself for what you are: eternal awareness infinitely connected to all that is, not a riddle to be figured out. Problems arise when you think an unpleasant feeling or character trait is permanent—which it never is. It only lasts as long as you insist on reinforcing its existence by thinking about it and holding on to it. If you think you're not in control of your thoughts, who do you think is? You have the power and the wisdom to let go of anything that you're willing to release. And all you have to do is . . . nothing. That's what's great about undoing. I've had students let go of and dissolve huge issues that had haunted their lives for years right in the middle of yoga class with no effort on my part or theirs. Something happens when the mind gets quiet and the body's energy begins to flow. The automatic release of negativity and baggage is a by-product of a quiet mind. And the result? Inner peace.

⚔ FINDING THE DIVINE WITHIN ⚔ (LATEX GLOVES NOT NECESSARY)

If the doors of perception were cleansed, everything would appear to man as it is, infinite.
—William Blake, *The Marriage of Heaven and Hell*

·→═◑═←·

There's nowhere to go for the truth, there's no one to pay, there's nothing to do. You can only undo all that is not true. And then you discover that truth was with you all along, concealed by everything false. That which is everlasting is just underneath everything that's temporary. And that which is divine is hiding behind everything that is mundane. Ever play hide-and-seek? In the same way, life is like a game, or play (*leela*). You must endeavor to find the truth and the divine in everything.

God concealed and God revealed are ways that yogis often describe the play of consciousness in the world. Everything is God everywhere all the time. But some things seem more obviously God than others. When you watch a beautiful sunset, that's obviously God. It would be considered God revealed. It's a little more of a challenge to see that a war zone with bullets flying and people screaming and dying is God, too. That would be considered God concealed. Compassion, love, or any genuine celebration of life is an example of God revealed. So even though it's all God, the yogis acknowledge that in duality, some things seem more like God than others. There are elements of the world that appear to be more of an expression of the perfection of God, of love and bliss, than others.

While an enlightened master sees that everything is God, given an option of the experience of God concealed or God revealed, there's usually a preference toward God revealed—love, compassion, freedom, bliss, truth—you get the picture.

God revealed is a little taste of the infinite, but so is God concealed; it just requires an able eye to see it. Yogis say that there's a big picture—and it's huge. An individual can only see a tiny little piece of this big picture. So you might look at your tiny piece and think, "What the hell is this? This doesn't look like anything! This looks like nonsense, fear, pain!" But when you see it in the context of the huge, enormous, gigantic, *big* picture, it all makes sense. Aha! Through love, compassion, surrender, allowing, forgiveness, joy, and other aspects of God revealed, you get a tiny glimpse of the big picture. But if you're stuck in a world where God is concealed through resistance, anger, hatred, violence, loathing, and so on, you're stuck with those little tidbits of the big picture that don't look like much.

What about experiences that seem like God revealed at first but later reveal themselves as God concealed? The drug heroin, for example, induces deep peace for some people—at first. Then it slowly ruins your entire life by destroying your body, depleting your finances, and, of course, requiring larger and larger doses to make you feel normal. Any recovering user will tell you the same story. This is true of many elements in the world. The yogis say these aspects of worldly life are like poison honey. The first symptom might be sweet, but the end is bitter.

Spiritual life is like a medicinal herb: bitter in the beginning, sweet in the end. Becoming conscious can initially be challenging. But once you get rolling, your life becomes peaceful, blissful, and much sweeter for your efforts.

How can a yogi experience God revealed all the time? God is what you are. The more you can let go of excessive thinking, the more you'll experience it. To reveal the God energy that you are, accept each moment. Acknowledge each moment as sacred. Don't resist what is. Look past the appearance through to the God just underneath.

Many yoga students are able to attain beautiful states of peace in yoga class, especially at the deeply relaxing end in shavasana. They experience God revealed when they feel happy and light, bliss pulsing through their bodies. But the moment they walk through the door and back into the real world, they get sucked back into the outward chaos of their lives and the inward chaos of their minds (God concealed). *Pick up the kids from school, is the husband happy? Massage at six, make sure the business is running smoothly, do I have enough money? I want to be single, I want a relationship, are my kids smart enough? My mother's in the hospital,* and on and on and on. This kind of activity could continue for the rest of your life, accelerating and picking up momentum like an avalanche. It can drive you insane or it can provoke inner surrender.

What's going to happen is going to happen. You can do what you can about it, but compulsive thought will only make it worse. Why not let go? If it succeeds in blissing you out at the end of yoga class, why not try it in your life? Do what you can and release the rest.

Your life is perfect as it is. Every aspect is exactly as it should be, pointing you precisely in the direction you're meant to go. Whether you're able to see it this way or not depends on how resistant you are to what is. Whether you can see it as God revealed or God concealed is a result of your point of view. What might seem like problems may actually be invitations for change. To reside as love, joy, compassion, stillness, and grace is to reside as the divine within and without. And this is the true yoga.

INNER YOGA

What does conflict do to you? Are you pushed toward complacency and depression, or do you feel pushed toward enhanced alertness and presence? If you could choose, which one would you prefer? Can you choose?

⊰ KARMA YOGA ⊱

Service which is rendered without joy helps neither the one who serves nor the served,
but all pleasures and possessions pale into nothingness before service
which is rendered in a spirit of joy.
—Mahatma Gandhi

◦───◉───◦

Once you realize that you and the world are perfect as they are, you won't feel guilty finding a rock in the woods to sit on in silence for the rest of your life. Many yogis have done that. In India, faced with an arranged marriage, a life of family drama, and the mundane, materialistic world, lots of people choose to put on the orange robes of a renunciate and seek a deeper truth. In the jungles of India, the caves have been filled with truth seekers for thousands of years. Many go to these caves, sit down in front of a fire, eat berries picked in the forest, realize their enlightenment, and never ever leave. It's a beautiful and acceptable life. By maintaining that energy and not sinking back into unconsciousness, you can become a silent part of evolution. By not polluting the world with worries and conflict, you are instantly doing the world a great service. The love and bliss that cave dwellers emanate ripples through the world, helping everyone in it. But it's not that easy for everyone. Some of us don't have a cave nearby. Some of us have jobs in office buildings and pets to feed.

It's easy to still the mind temporarily: surfing, a hard workout, sexing yourself silly, eating yourself into a coma. But full bliss won't reveal itself to you in a lasting way from a quick fix like this. Real, lasting inner peace is not a product of brief stillness in the ego-mind. Real meditation is not just an hour a day; it's twenty-four hours a day and becomes everything you do. When every action is performed with full attention, in a way that doesn't solidify the illusion of a psychological identification with the ego-mind, you are meditating, merging, practicing yoga every second.

To bring this practice into your day-to-day work involves the practice of karma yoga. Karma yoga is to work selflessly, dissolving the ego and letting the divine do the work. This constant meditation and service is a very high practice. By not feeding the ego, by really focusing on what you're doing, and becoming aware of yourself as a vehicle for the divine, you are freeing yourself in every moment.

It's not you working a grueling, ten-hour day, it's the divine working through what seems to be you. When you take yourself out of the equation and realize you're not doing anything, it is being done through you, it's a real load off the old back. Life gets easier. Instead of feeling drained and tired from the pressure of making a living, it's actually really fun and energy producing. It's only when the ego-mind thinks you're doing everything that you can build a story around it and get exhausted and stressed out. The truth is that you don't do anything, you just *allow* work to be done by the divine, through you. And that's where freedom comes in. If you think you're doing the work, you have to deal with the duality, the repercussions, the karma.

In karma yoga, you're not the doer. Even if you believe you are the doer, you're not. You used to believe in Santa Claus, so how reliable are beliefs? Life is happening through you. When you get this, you might be able to truly enjoy work. You may be conscious of thoughts arising, but you are not those thoughts. You are the consciousness that is aware of the thoughts arising. You may be aware of work happening, but it's not being done by you, it's coming through you. You are the consciousness aware of the work.

True karma yoga is the divine serving the divine. Where you see a problem, that is your calling to work. Mother Teresa practiced karma yoga, although she probably didn't call it that. All she did was work and help, to the point that the person doing this work disappeared. She became her work. True karma yoga is not done for the good feeling of being a helper, it is done for its own sake. Everything happens—walking, digestion, smiling, breathing—and is there a you that has to do it? No. It just happens. Inner peace happens, and you don't have to be Mother Teresa to know it's not you doing it. Work can also happen this way.

To let your work—whatever it may be—work through you produces no karma, good or bad. If you—as the ego—have saved the world, that's good karma. Congratulations! You've saved the world! And although it's better than bad karma, it still involves an ego. Don't be fooled; good karma is also binding. Yogis call it the golden chain, because you're still chained down to thoughts and identities, even though your chains are the best on the market and made of gold. In this world of duality, what is good for one may be bad for another. Most of us can't see the big picture in its entirety. The executioner might think he's doing a service by hanging a man who he thinks is evil. But what happens when that man is proved innocent after his death? What happens to the well-meaning family of the executed? What happens to this do-gooder and his service then? Do our puny little minds really know so much? Does one individual mind really know more than the infinite power that creates and enlivens the universe? I doubt it. So doing good deeds for ego gratification won't do much good for you or anyone else in the grand scheme of things.

To serve without the ego, only to be the channel through which the divine operates, is true karma yoga. The reward of selfless service? The joy of selfless service and inner peace. It's only from this point of surrender that you can actually do the world any good. But it's also perfectly fine to sit on a rock in complete bliss for the rest of your life. That's also a substantial contribution.

To truly practice karma yoga is to become a saint in the eyes of the yogis. It's an extremely advanced practice. You can try it in short spurts at first. You don't have to change much, just your point of view. As your perception of the world shifts, don't be too surprised if the world starts to shift as well. Those who practice karma yoga report the experience of limitless energy. Where they may have only been able to work non-stop for four hours at a time, by getting the ego out of the way and allowing work to happen through them, they are able to work for sixteen hours without any symptom of exhaustion. Creative ideas flow steadily through them. And as they work, there's a feeling of life force increasing, of working with love and an open heart. This is not achieved through effort, but through getting out of the way. It's a very natural state.

You may not be ready for this kind of transformation. Then again, maybe you are, but you're too distracted to realize it. There's a famous yogi story that when you're a little child, you get lots of toys in your playroom. As long as you're happily playing with these toys, your mother will leave you there and go about her business. It's only when you get tired of these toys, when they no longer satisfy you, and you scream and cry for your mother, that she will come to you. The same is true of God awareness. As long as you are contented with your distractions, God will not come into your experience. When you are no longer satisfied with the little pleasures of the world and your soul screams for something real, then God awareness happens to you. Inner peace happens. And once inner peace happens to you, you're forever changed.

TIPS FOR REMEMBERING WHO YOU REALLY ARE

❋ You are not your identity. You are not your history, your story, your ancestors, your relatives, your job, your house, your car, your spouse, your hobbies, your children, or your shoes. In this moment, and in every moment, you are freedom. Don't forget.

❋ Be motivated by your fears and resistances. Look at them like you would a hallucination. What's real?

❋ Truly be of service. Live without expectations and work without schemes. Lose yourself in service to others with no thought of reward. Watch what happens—this deepens your understanding of who you are and the experience of the power of the universal source working through you.

SUPPLEMENTS TO ENHANCE YOUR DAILY GRIND

Green tea extract is both stimulating and relaxing. It contains caffeine, but not nearly as much as coffee or black tea. I'd recommend it as a replacement for whatever you normally caffeinate yourself with in the morning (if you do). It also contains powerful antioxidants.

Vinpocetine is a brain stimulant. It's known to increase blood flow to the brain. If you're going to use your brain, you may as well use as much of it as you can.

L-theanine is an amino acid naturally found in green tea. It has a tranquilizing effect on the brain, relaxing it without shutting it down. It promotes clarity and enhances the ability to learn and remember. In Japan, it's commonly added to chewing gum and soft drinks to heighten performance in the workplace.

POSTURES TO EXPAND YOUR AWARENESS OF WHO YOU ARE

Become aware of the energy that animates your body. Direct and move this energetic awareness into these poses. If your energy's in the pose, your body and mind will follow.

Try something the mind says you won't be able to do. What does the mind know? Apparently, not much.

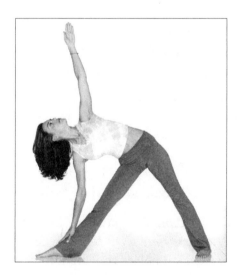

TRIKONASANA (TRIANGLE)

Standing with your feet 3 to 3½ feet apart, turn your right foot out about 90 degrees. Turn your left foot in slightly. With your legs straight, raise your arms up sideways to shoulder height, extending straight out, palms facing down. As you exhale, reach your right arm out over your right leg, allowing your body to follow, until your right hand reaches your right leg. Place your hand on your knee, shin, ankle, or on the floor next to your right foot. Extend your left arm up toward the ceiling in line with your left shoulder. Look toward your left hand, and roll your upper body open and back in alignment with your legs. Stay in this pose for 30 seconds to a minute.

Eventually come back to the starting position, reverse your feet, and do the other side.

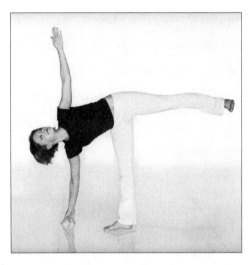

ARDHA CHANDRASANA (HALF MOON)

Standing, spread your feet about 3½ feet apart. Extend your arms to your sides at shoulder level. Turn your right foot out 90 degrees, bend your right knee, lean to the right, and place your right fingertips on the floor 6 inches to the right of your right foot. At the same time, lift your left leg off the ground until it's parallel to the floor. Your arms should be straight and perpendicular to the floor, parallel to the walls. Open your hips and shoulders. Look up, down, or toward the facing wall. Hold for about 30 seconds, then repeat on the left side.

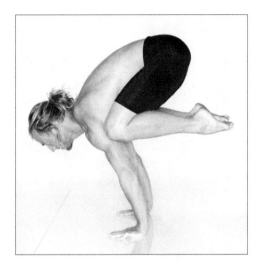

KAKASANA (CROW)

From a squatting position, place your hands on the floor in front of you. Lean all of your weight onto your hands, keeping your arms bent. Place your knees on your upper arms almost in your armpits, and slowly lift your feet off the floor. Balance and look straight ahead.

PLAYLIST SUGGESTIONS

1. "The Wind" · Cat Stevens
2. "Shape of My Heart" · Sting
3. "Presence of the Lord" · Blind Faith
4. "Stuck in a Moment" · U2
5. "How Little It Matters" · Frank Sinatra
6. "Do What I Gotta Do" · Donnell Jones
7. "When We Get By" · D'Angelo
8. "Oh Gosh" · Donovan

If you cannot find the truth right where you are,
where else do you expect to find it?

—Dogen Zenji

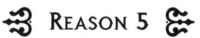 **REASON 5**

YOU CAN CHANGE YOUR WORLD

The morning of September 11th, I was at home getting ready to teach my morning yoga class when the news reached me. I immediately began fielding phone calls from terrified, sobbing friends, and then I began trying to make my own calls to friends in New York. I drove to the yoga studio just in case one or two people showed up, although I assumed no one would show up at all. When I walked into the yoga room at Maha, to my astonishment, the class was packed. The room was full of frazzled, freaked-out yogis ready to practice. We went through a normal asana practice, ending in meditation. The focus on yoga practice throughout was remarkable, all things considered. I spoke to friends of mine who are teachers in other cities, and this was not an isolated phenomenon.

There's very little we can do by the time the horrors of the world show up on our doorstep. But yoga practice is one of the few activities that can focus the mind, open the heart, and reveal inner peace in the face of external chaos. That morning, many people who hadn't allowed themselves to process their feelings around the violent destruction they'd witnessed started breaking down and sobbing in class. Inner peace doesn't mean stuffing emotions away; it means allowing yourself to feel what is without suppression—a beautiful and very healing practice.

Practicing yoga in times of intense drama and tragedy won't change what has already happened in the world. It may not undo a slap, a gunshot, or a war, but it can stop a cycle. When someone hits you, a natural reaction is to hit back out of anger. Then you get hit again, then you hit again, and on and on. But what if after the first insult, you don't react unconsciously? What if you just watch your impulse to react without indulging in it or acting it out? Instead of a gut reaction, you can access your most effective, peace-invoking reaction from a clear, focused point of view.

Some yogis say that the world is a kind of training ground, that it's riddled with conflict for a good reason: to push you toward that which is beyond all duality. The chaos of the world can indeed be a great motivator for cultivating inner peace. And your own inner peace can be a great inspiration for the rest of the world.

⊰ WORLD PEACE THROUGH INNER PEACE ⊱

As is the human body, so is the cosmic body.
As is the human mind, so is the cosmic mind.
As is the microcosm, so is the macrocosm.
As is the atom, so is the universe.
—The Upanishads

I once asked a very wise old yogi in India how he came to choose his path. He told me very openly that it was due to his mother's influence, and from his point of view, although not yogic in the obvious ways, she was a very high yogini. Before he was born, this yogi's mother had lived in the northern part of India. Northern India has been occupied, conquered, converted, and battled over more often than anyone would care to mention. This yogi's mother lived in a little mountain village rather precariously positioned geographically; whether armies came from the north, south, east, or west, whether coming or going, attacking or defending, they would invariably pass through her village. When she was a child, the people of her village could hear the armies approaching from miles away. The men of the house were usually off fighting, so the women were left to fend for themselves. They would grab their children and hide in cupboards, trunks—anywhere they might not be noticed—and with good reason: Armies tended to view other people as objects, as strategic obstacles. After being robbed of their food supplies, women were often raped, killed, or otherwise abused.

One day when she was about ten years old, this yogi's mother, Radha, was baking bread with her mother. They heard an army approaching. The marching made the furniture quiver and shudder as the pounding of the soldiers' boots drew nearer and nearer. All the women of the village ran to their hiding places, but not little Radha. She remained in her mother's kitchen and continued kneading and rolling the dough. Her mother called for her, but Radha quietly refused to hide. She'd had enough of running and hiding in her life. She made a very profound decision: She decided she'd rather die than spend another three days hiding in a dark, cold closet. Was it Radha's innocence that made her fearless? Her youth? Or was she just wise enough to know that she'd rather die than spend another moment possessed by fear?

With all the other women hidden away, Radha baked loaf after loaf all by herself. And when the army arrived, she went outside and greeted the troops with freshly baked breads and sweets. She treated them as though they were her missing brothers, uncles, and father. Instead of being full of fear, she was full of love—or full of God, as the yogi would say. The soldiers were won over by this fearless ten-year-old, and they ate the bread, suddenly timid as church mice from the brave love of this child. Radha continued in this way every time a new army passed through, and she was always left unscathed. The women who hid in the cupboards were astonished that no harm came to this little girl. They scolded her and called her crazy. But Radha's son, now a very wise yogi, understands what happened. Love is disarming. Radha transformed the atmosphere of fear and hate into an atmosphere of love and grace. Instead of seeing her as an enemy—as a foreigner—the passing armies saw in her the love of their own mothers, sisters, and wives. Gracious love, generous love, conscious love, instantly transforms you into everyone's family. Love transforms the *us* and the *them* into just *us*. In Radha's lifetime, the wars never stopped—that little town was technically and politically part of many different countries and controlled by many different leaders. Radha lived in a town constantly under siege, but she made sure she was always at peace.

What makes war? Conflict. Where does conflict come from? Conflict begins as a thought or a feeling: wanting land, wanting power, wanting money, wanting control—just wanting. Where does wanting come from? Wanting comes from dissatisfaction.

If war starts as a thought, how can you fight it? How do you defeat an invisible force? The seed in the ego-mind that will eventually grow into physical enemies and active physical conflict is physically intangible. You can't shoot, wrestle, or poison the spark that ignites all negativity in the world: negative thoughts. If your freedom were threatened physically, if someone tried to tie your hands and feet, you could endeavor to defend yourself, grab the rope away from your attacker, fight, or negotiate your way to liberation. When a country's freedom is jeopardized, the army is rallied to fend off any such menace. These physical offenders are physically defended. But how do you defend yourself against the root of all violence and despair in the world, the invisible attacks, negative thoughts, emotions, drama, and inner turmoil?

Start by focusing on your own personal peace. Negativity would like to lure you into a negative state. Your ego-mind can build a case against anything or anyone available. Your best defense is to acknowledge the negative ego-mind without empowering thoughts by believing them to be true or acting on them. This way, the negativity of the ego-mind weakens. For example, do you ever notice your mind producing the following thoughts: "Nothing ever goes right for me. I'll never be happy" or "Everyone's out to get me. This whole office is against me." It's possible to observe these thoughts but not believe them. Realize it's the ego-mind and don't become its puppet. Don't let the ego pull you into an emotional downward spiral. It's like a bully trying to get a rise out of you—don't be sucked into its clever provocations. You're better off walking away or looking the bully straight in the eye without fear. When you engage with negativity and acknowledge it as real and important, you empower and strengthen it. If you allow it to come up, but face it head-on with love, you will disarm it. The ego will lose its power over you. By remaining alert and aware of thought streams as potentially misleading companions, you are practicing very advanced yoga: watching the mind.

The world's problems aren't collective; they're personal. There is no political solution, religion, world diet, or business plan that is going to pacify the world's conflicts in one fell swoop. The world's problems are your problems. What can you do toward world peace? Find out who you really are. Be the change that you want to see.

⋺ THE WORLD AS LEELA ⋊

If you listen to the news for five minutes, you might be suckered into believing that the list of disasters they're telling you about are shocking—full of first-time-ever occurrences. It's the aim of the media—whether they know it or not—to excite you, engage you, and frighten you. But if you look at their reports objectively and ignore the panicked tone of the newscaster (live from the disaster site!) you may be able to detect a pattern: Humans are humans, and as long as we are all sleepwalking, history will repeat itself.

The yogic approach to the world is quite different from what you're probably used to. Instead of being repeatedly shocked by the atrocities of mankind, yogis accept them completely. A yogi saint sees war and conflict (and everything else) as *leela*: the play of the divine. Like a company of actors, God is playing all the roles—creating the world as we know it.

Religions often preach about good and evil. Yogis say it's all grace. It's grace that the flower blossoms, but it's also grace that makes the flower wilt and die. Everything is divine. Yes, wars come, and then wars go, but from the yogic point of view, the world has been a play of good and bad longer than history can record. There have been short periods of peace and harmony in societies, but these moments are like specks of dust on a vast stage of war, hunger, and unrest. It's the exception to learn about peaceful, happy civilizations—it's far more common to hear about the violence, greed, and upheaval. Just take a look at a history book: War is the one constant activity.

So why is everyone so surprised when violence and insanity happen? It's much more surprising when they don't happen. And yet, as the state of the world grows more furious and desperate, the urge toward change, compassion, and love is also heightened. More people are waking up from their unconscious negativity and searching for deeper meaning and connection. As frightening as it may seem, it is a fortunate time to be alive. Now more than ever, the incentive to awaken is tremendous.

The politics of your very own family may be just as nutty, if not more nutty, than the politics of the world. How much screaming and distress can happen when a teenage boy violates his teenage sister's privacy? The sky's the limit. Anger, rage, and even violence can be provoked by the tiniest transgressions. The primitive, reptilian mind-set dominating the behavior of the vast majority of people lashes out and tries to kill what it doesn't understand. That includes life, love, and other beautiful mysteries of existence.

How can you think that world peace can ever happen if you can't make peace with yourself? There seem to be so many good reasons to be neurotic and stressed out. There's always intense chaos and violence somewhere. The challenge the yogi faces is this: What do you do about it? What is your reaction? There are wars happening all over the world, people are starving needlessly, most governments are corrupt, criminals roam the streets, your local police force probably has dirty cops, there are broken stoplights causing untold driving hazards, your own parents might be manipulative and operating with a questionable mind-set, your children could be caught up in strange, new adolescent societies. There's always some source of chaos waiting, wanting, wishing to suck you into its fury like a hurricane. What do you do? It's not always possible or advisable to ignore big issues, problems, and dramas. But getting involved can often mean being consumed by—or worse, transformed into—the ugliness of the monster you're out to conquer.

As within, so without. You want world peace? You must become that which you seek. You must become conscious. How many people does it take to achieve world peace? One. You.

⊰ THE WORLD AS A CATALYST ⊱

If the purpose of life is transcendence and enlightenment, can you imagine a world perfectly designed for your evolution? In a way, this world is. The action and reaction of everyday living sets in motion an unstoppable chain of events that all point in the same direction—if you're paying attention. In every moment exists the opportunity to be awake, and every moment can be your perfect teacher. It is a yoga practice to see the world as a catalyst for rousing you from the complacency of unconsciousness. And sometimes the universe just won't take no for an answer.

As the world is becoming more absurd, if you can no longer shut out the chaos, the odds become stacked in your favor toward realization. You can view the strange, modern conditions of the world as positive and negative, or you can see them as simply heightened. The state of the world is the state of the world. What you do with it is up to you.

What I'm talking about here is beyond the normal mechanics of living. It's beyond voting for the politician you think will be the most effective leader, beyond consuming wisely, beyond purchasing ecologically conscious products, beyond recycling, beyond driving a hybrid or low-pollution vehicle. It's great to do everything you can to be helpful and positive, but beyond your actions, the world will go on. There will be things that you can't control. You may live in a home that is run on solar energy from panels you installed yourself, and yet, an oil spill or a nuclear meltdown may still happen. Despite your efforts, its repercussions could even directly affect you, contaminating your water supply or radiating the ground you live on. What can you do about the aspects of existence that are out of your control? You can worry and complain until you induce early death from a heart attack, or these elements can be your most potent teachers.

Our fears and anxieties exist so that we can transcend them. When the world comes blasting through our safe little corners in the form of politics, war, and other worldly dysfunctions, we are left with no recourse. There's nothing left to do. The choices are simple: Resist and be miserable; get stuck in thoughts, criticisms, and relentless mental complaining; or accept what is and relinquish the fantasy that we have control over that which is uncontrollable. Use circumstance to see past the world to the ultimate truth.

Our deepest, most primal fear is the fear of death, a topic I'll cover at length in Reason 6. Death is going to happen to everybody at one point or another. Sure, you can be cryogenically frozen to be defrosted at a better time, but that is not a means of escaping the fear of dying. In fact, it empowers your fear of death with the hope of escape. What happens if a war interrupts your frozen slumber? The world can pop in at the most inconvenient moments. There is no real escape from fear. Never getting on an airplane won't eradicate your fear of flying. You won't have to deal with it as long as you don't climb into a jet, but whether or not you ever fly, you will still have your fear. Going through fears, not avoiding them, will dissolve them.

There is a very famous Indian yogi, Sri Ramana Maharshi, who had a rare, complete, spontaneous awakening at the age of sixteen. He was in his small bedroom just after school when he suddenly felt a powerful and overwhelming fear of death. He lay down on the floor of his room and began to go through the motions of dying. He stopped his breath and he imagined that he was dead. He imagined his body being carried to the cremation grounds. He thought, *Now I am dead. Where have I gone? What am I now? Beyond this body, what am I? Who is it that is aware of being dead?* It was then that he realized who he was, and he became Self-realized and enlightened. He left his house, relinquished his identity, and wandered to a holy temple at the foot of a mountain called Arunachala. He sat at the foot of this mountain in absolute bliss and total silence without moving for several years. A local monk would put enough food in his mouth every day to sustain his body. Later Ramana would wander up to the caves of this mountain and sit there in silence. He never left Arunachala. Truth seekers from all over the world would come just to sit in his presence. When he was silent they would bask in the powerful, blissful energy pouring from his being. When he finally began to speak, more than fifteen years after his initial awakening, they came for his words of tremendous love, insight, and wisdom. Seekers continue to pilgrimage to this mountain, although Ramana has long since left this earth. That awakened energy is still palpable where he sat in meditation in his temple and on his mountain. I've been there many times, and I can confirm that the energy is as powerful, alive, and tangible as sticking your thumb in an electric socket.

Ramana went through his deepest, darkest fear and it woke him up to the truth of his being. It's rare for it to happen in just a moment as it did for him. When it does, it can take some time to adjust to the new point of view. It's like going from 0 to 150 miles an hour in five seconds. When enlightenment happens this quickly, it's often followed by a long period of silence—inner and outer quiet. Spontaneous awakenings are rare; enlightenment is usually not so easy, nor is it so fast. But going through your deepest, darkest fears will wake you up to the truth of your being, if not in an instant, then gradually. By watching the mind with vigilance, seeking the truth about yourself tirelessly, and allowing and going through your fears as they arise, you'll find your level of awareness subtly heightens and heightens. When enlightenment is attained gradually, it's integrated into daily life gently, naturally.

Waking up to the ultimate reality is not something that can be done for you by a priest, an energy healer, an acupuncturist, or a chiropractor. The undoing of collective conditioning starts with your own individual mastery of discernment. When you feel fear, when you feel any kind of resistance, look into the heart of the matter and ask yourself, "What is this? What am I? What am I really afraid of? Who is afraid? Who is angry? Who is feeling?" Return to the essence of who you are, that perfect awareness of being. Don't blame the world or the people and situations in your life for what they are. Become aware of what is within and what is outside of your control. Surrender to the moment, allow what is to be as it is, and look to yourself for your reactions. By correcting yourself, you are making a tremendous contribution to the collective peace on this planet. Let the world bring your unconsciousness out of you, and when you become aware of it, allow it and release it. Let it go and be free.

⊰ ELIMINATE YOUR POLITICS ⊱

In order to seek our own direction, one must simplify the mechanics
of ordinary, everyday life.
—**Plato**

→✦←

If you want to go through life completely stressed out, full of fear, or in anticipation of looming disaster, I would recommend staying closely tuned in to the politics of the world. What better way to gather resources to fuel the neurotic, obsessive mind? One hour with a newspaper can provide enough material for lots of anxiety, endless conversation, two sessions a week with your therapist, extraneous thought activity, and even nightmares. If this is what you're into, by all means, go for broke. On the other hand, if you're interested in feeling bliss or even having a good yoga practice, it might be time to consider giving the TV a vacation and letting your newspaper subscription expire.

I'm not saying it's a bad thing to know what's going on in the world, because it isn't. The trouble comes once the information reaches the compulsively thinking mind. What do you think will happen? Hardwired to troubleshoot, the unruly mind has its tricks. Reports of chaos, violence, and destruction feed the obsessive, worrying, negative habits of the mind, reinforcing compulsive thinking. Behaviors get fixed by constant repetition—and so do anxious thoughts. You can't worry or think your way to inner peace. When you learn to stop obsessing, to stop chewing on the same old ideas and emotions over and over again, that's when you find some peace. The idea is not to stop thinking permanently, the idea is to be able to have a choice: Do you feel like thinking right now or not? Will thinking help you recognize the perfection of this beautiful moment? Is your current thought something you want on your mind right now or not? Is your amazing, perfect life slipping by while you're caught up in thoughts of the future, the past, fantasies, and calculations? Most people can't stop thinking if they want to. Thinking is an addiction, and thinking is a contraction of what you truly are. Thinking can be bondage. When it becomes your choice, to think or not to think—that is freedom.

When you think about world politics or debate world politics, often you're dealing with matters that aren't directly affecting you. In fact, you may not ever see the people you're shouting your opinions about. There's nothing wrong with caring, but what are you caring about? What you read in the news or see on television is put into context by the reporter, by the news agency, and by the filters of your own mind. The media is often distorted—skewed to present a slanted and reactionary viewpoint designed to incite an emotional response. By the time a situation gets to you, it isn't even close to what you would have witnessed if you'd been there yourself. So what are you really thinking about and reacting to? Other compulsive thinkers' thoughts? Who really knows? It all just distracts your attention from the true issues: Who are you? Why are you here? What is life? What is death? What is real?

If you're serious about inner peace, it's advisable to take a break from over-intellectualizing—or intellectualizing at all—events that you hear about from the media. Until you are in control of whether or not you think, don't torture yourself. Get your own world in order first, then, if you must, check out other people's dramas. Recovering alcoholics don't spend their free time in bars.

I know many people (myself included) who have taken months and years away from television and newspapers, and when they tuned back in, they were amazed that not much had changed in the world: Wars were still happening, natural disasters, leaders coming and going, governments wrestling for control and power. The difference is that when you're watching the news as it's happening, there's an element of spontaneity. You feel as though this horrible event is special because it's happening right this second. When you look at the news of the past, what seemed so urgent and shocking in the moment just slips in perfectly with the long list of other disastrous events; the emotional urgency is gone. The only difference between the news of now and the past is the advent of technology, which allows violence to happen on a larger scale. More people have the ability to harm more people. Other than that, it's just the same old story: Man is acting out his unconsciousness.

Most of what the media has to offer is basically gossip. If you're really not involved in something personally, if you're not an element of a matter you're discussing, it's a kind of mental masturbation. Why talk about something you're not involved with? You may as well be saying, "I heard Becky's cheating on Philip. But then you never know, because I heard that from Rita. And I heard from someone else that Rita spreads rumors." It's senseless mind noise. If you want peace, turn it off.

INNER YOGA

1. As an experiment, try to avoid the media for one day. For one day, don't watch any television, don't read the newspaper, and don't read magazines.

2. If you have successfully avoided the media for one day, try it for one week.

3. If you have gone for one week, try it for a month. Notice how life has an ease and harmony to it that you may have overlooked before. Now sell your TV and use the newspaper only to line your birdcage!

⊰ YOUR OWN PRIVATE POLITICS ⊱

Unfortunately, politics don't end when you turn off the news. Politics find their way into your city, town, house, marriage, siblings, children, and so on. Constant negotiations, projections of the future, and the millions of ways people try to control one another for their own benefit weave an utterly vain web of worry and compulsive thinking: "Well, if I do that, then she'll do this." "If I wear that, then they'll think this."

To carefully politic your way through life is a surefire way to work your nervous system into a breakdown. Politics are all about wanting control. But if the thing you're wanting to control is impossible to control—for example, any person, place, or thing other than yourself—you're certainly in for a rocky ride. People pleasers have it the worst: It takes immense thought and energy to get the superficial approval of someone else. And when you get it—if you get it—that approval simply fans the fire to look for more superficial approval. And that's not really going to take you anywhere except exhaustion avenue.

If you're seeking the approval of someone else, thinking that will make you happy, or if you're trying to control someone else, thinking that will make you happy, you're just setting yourself up for a fall. *All expectation creates disappointment.* To think that happiness and peace are anywhere other than within yourself is a common, yet painful mistake. You may as well be a leaf in the wind blowing hither and thither. First, get centered in your own true nature. Then, whether you're living in the Taj Mahal or above your parents' garage or on a park bench, you will be living the life of a yogi king. The most valuable thing in the world is the peace that you have inside of you. Once you have that, all doors open to you. To the mind that's still, the whole universe surrenders.

Politics begin with you. You can see tense, stressful personal situations in families, businesses, clubs, and schools comparable in political complexity to trade embargos and hostage situations. If you let these politics swallow you up and become your identity, I can promise you it will be a never-ending struggle. At all times it's important to stay focused on the whole picture—the divine—not the shallow end of the pool. That doesn't mean you have to stay alone for the rest of your life or remove yourself from every conflict-ridden situation. It just means you become aware of what's really going on around you. Although a situation may be dreadful, it's also temporary and perfect. In any given moment there are several levels from which you can be aware of your experience. It's the difference between being consumed by a situation and being able to function in your situation while maintaining awareness of the bigger picture. And in that awareness is freedom—the freedom to be without drama and the freedom to be without the suffering that always goes with it.

INNER YOGA

1. Do you ever try to control other people? (Hint: Yes!) Look deeply into your experience. If you find that you do want to control other people, do you think you could let go of that desire? How do you think you would feel if you let go of wanting control?

2. How long can you go without thinking? Try it right now. . . . Okay, try again.

3. Try focusing on one thing at a time. Focus on the task at hand. If your mind wanders, watch it, notice where it goes. Stay alert and constantly bring it back to the task at hand.

4. Just to notice how wild and uncontrolled the mind is, sit down for two minutes and watch the breath go in and out. Stay absolutely present with the mind. This is an ancient and beautiful meditation. It's simple and yet more difficult than you might think. But don't think, just watch.

⊰ LOST IN THE CHAOS? ⊱

Your trials did not come to punish you, but to awaken you—to make you realize that you are part of Spirit and that just behind the spark of your life is the flame of infinity.
—Paramahansa Yogananda

The state of the world can seem overwhelmingly complex and frightening. The mind reels. It's amazingly easy to get sucked into mental chaos, get used to it, and stay there for the rest of your life, thinking that's all there is. But contrary to popular belief, it's not outer chaos that's the problem. Stress and worry come from the ego-mind's desire to organize, categorize, and control the outside world. It's not the world, it's the thinking that creates the issue.

India is one of the most outwardly chaotic places in the universe. When I first made the journey, it was almost like visiting another planet. Cows, pigs, and dogs are everywhere, the air is full of dust, everything is covered in a layer of dirt, very little that's mechanical works. People—normal, middle-class, working people, not homeless people—lie down and take naps on the sidewalk when they get sleepy. A cacophony of bells, car horns, people yelling and praying, music playing, and motors running fills the air perpetually. It's almost impossible for me to describe India because it's such an extraordinary place: The appearance is chaotic and seems like a delirious dream, and yet the feeling I have when I'm there is one of utter peace and harmony with the universe. It's almost inconceivable until you experience it for yourself. What I find exceptional about the people who live there is their rare capacity to embrace intense chaos—or what would seem to be chaos to a visitor's eye.

On the road in India, whether you're in a car, taxi, or bus, you have to participate in the most dangerous form of the game chicken ever known to mankind. Passing is legal anywhere, anytime. There are no lanes. I'm not exaggerating when I say that many, many times I have found myself in the back of a taxi moving at well over seventy-five miles per hour going directly toward a car or truck coming from the other direction, about to meet head-on in what could easily be the end of my life in this body. Fortunately, the drivers have reflexes like Olympians, and just a split second before there's about to be a very large explosion that involves bits of me flying to opposite ends of the road, both drivers swerve and fly past each other with less than an inch between them. This ritual is performed well over ten times in one twenty-minute drive. So you can imagine the deep surrender that happens just from being driven around. You can either be miserable or surrender to the moment. Everyone drives that way, and if your driver didn't drive that way, you wouldn't get anywhere. You're forced to come to terms with the fact that you're not in control of whether you live or die, especially while you're on the road in India. Who knew you could be driven toward enlightenment?

What's veritably exceptional are the calm, smiling faces of the speed racer drivers. These fast-paced, supercongested roads would push any normal U.S. urbanite beyond the point of self-control to a frantic state of deadly road rage. In India, they just drive along at breakneck speeds while remaining happy as larks and calmer than most massage therapists. There are no posted speed limits, no highway patrol, no driving age, rarely a center divider, no lanes, shoulders are fair game, and usually no stoplights or stop signs. Add to the equation pedestrians and cows freely roaming the roads, and in some areas large swarms of pigs or camels can also be spotted gallivanting amid the 80-mile-per-hour rush of vehicles.

I think it has something to do with surrender and acceptance. Nothing is expected to be any other way than as it is. There is intense outer chaos, and yet beautiful inner peace. Because there are no rules, no one can break them. Everyone's just going where they're going. And because there's little or no traffic control, drivers stay very alert and there's no dependence on an outer source of authority. I know it's difficult to wrap the mind around, but it's true. After a taxi ride (if you survive), you can weather any challenge. It's a deep spiritual experience. Amidst pandemonium and disorder there can be an amazing inner surrender.

If you're going to get married in India, the first thing you have to do is consult a Vedic astrologer who determines the most auspicious date and time for the marriage ceremony to occur. This precise time is firmly adhered to without question or pause, whether it's two in the morning or four in the afternoon. So you may be peacefully dreaming the night away, when suddenly, at 3:00 A.M., you snap to your senses to the sound of Ricky Martin blasting through loudspeakers (they have the most powerful speakers in India), or bells ringing, or crowds cheering. Firecrackers are also very popular . . . and loud. The choices are clear: insanity and rage or inner surrender. What are you going to do? Stop a wedding party of two hundred from broadcasting Celine Dion for four square miles? I don't think so. So you let it go. It's happening and you allow it. Don't worry about it—make a pot of tea, or go join the wedding celebration, or put in your earplugs. In other words, be gracious and allow things to be as they are—especially if it's out of your hands (which it usually is)!

I was in line once at an enormous temple in Bombay. There were literally thousands of people filing through this ancient holy place. The woman in front of me was holding an infant, and in India it's common for babies to wear no diaper. All of a sudden, the baby started shooting out diarrhea. As poop flew through the air, the mom just held the baby out away from her—toward me—and let the child squirt all over the temple floor. They were right in front of me and I was definitely within firing range. What was I going to do? This was their way. The baby can't help it, there's no diaper, the mother couldn't understand me if I asked her to aim the baby's butt somewhere else because she speaks only Hindi. There was nothing I could do. The situation was all systems go—it was happening. I quickly moved away from the flying mess and felt grateful that I'd avoided a potential soiling. But then I looked down at my bare feet— you take your shoes off before you go into holy places in India—and I realized that this happened every day as thousands of people file through this place. It seemed I had separated myself from the poop, but I hadn't. It's everywhere. It turns into dust and it settles wherever it wants to. There's no escaping the chaos (or shit, as the case may be) that flies around this world. Inevitably, it's right where you are. Sometimes you just have to take a shallow breath and walk on. Or hold your nose and walk through it.

Inner surrender is the main thing. You can try to separate yourself as much as you want. You can work on attracting situations conducive to inner peace, but it's not really much of an accomplishment if you can maintain some semblance of tranquility in a climate-controlled, well-decorated, padded room. What happens when you're forced to walk from your front door to your car? Or visit relatives? Or go to the market? You just can't control everything and everyone. And how embarrassing is it to lose it and flip your lid at a parking attendant after you've spent twenty years at meditation practice? If you can't maintain your inner calm amidst chaos, you need more practice, because chaos is where you need it.

Yoga practice can give you a taste of deep inner peace, but there's no reason to limit your experience of bliss and a quiet mind to yoga class. When you're surrounded by your normal chaos, it can become a battle, but that's the most important time to practice what you learn in yoga. If you can stay aware of your mind's thoughts and re-actions, the outward chaos loses its power over you. This is an aspect of true freedom: unwavering peace despite the conditions of the world.

Unwavering peace might start in a silent forest on an untroubled rock near a placid lake, but you must learn to extend it into your world, into your daily life. That doesn't mean controlling or changing the world, it means loving the world and ac-cepting the world—and yourself—exactly as they are. If you want to change the world or yourself, and you are able to do so, do it! Surrender to that, be that, and do that. If not, learn to accept things as they are. Happiness arises from acceptance of yourself, others, the world, and this moment. Allow this moment to be as it is and feel the peace that is always waiting for you.

If you can be as you are where you are, great, but to be in internal combat with the world or yourself seems loony once you realize you have a choice.

INNER YOGA

The next time you're in a crowded, busy place, close your eyes and listen to the sound. Can you hear it as one sound instead of a collection of many, fragmented noises? Just listen to this sound, put all your attention on the sound. Do this for a minute or two. How does it make you feel?

⊰ **THE WORLD AS YOUR GURU** ⊱

If you gaze for long enough into the abyss, the abyss also gazes into you.
—**Friedrich Nietzsche,** *Beyond Good and Evil*

⋆⊷⊙⊶⋆

A guru doesn't have to be a stereotypical Indian guy shouting orders at you all the time (although sometimes that can help). The world works just as well. From the viewpoint of a realized yogi, the unpredictable world looks absolutely perfect just as it is. The magic of cause and effect takes everyone through exactly what they need to go through precisely when they need to go through it. The word *guru* translates from ancient Sanskrit to mean "that which brings you from darkness to light." It's a term that can be used to describe a human teacher, but it can also be used to describe anything that brings you into true awareness. If you see the phenomenal world as an expression of the divine, then you can also see it as your guru. And the more you see it this way, the more it will become such. You will be led and guided by the phenomenal world if you see it as your teacher. The world will reward you and the world will discipline you. It's as much one with the infinite as you are, and even if you can't see it this way, the world will still teach you.

It's possible to watch the politics of the world just as one watches thoughts in the mind. There's no need to empower a thought by believing it to be the ultimate reality. Similarly, there's no need to empower a disaster or political crisis as the ultimate reality. Acknowledge the world, watch the world, but know that it's constantly changing and that it's largely out of your control. Remain focused on that which doesn't change. Stay in this moment. It is always this moment. There's still a chance for a peaceful world and it begins with you. It begins right now. Every waking second is a chance to look past who you think you are right through to who you truly are.

TIPS FOR SUSTAINING INNER PEACE

❈ As long as there is inner conflict, history will repeat itself. A yogi's primary concern is the attainment of inner peace and bliss.

❈ The states of the world can push you toward complacency or enlightenment. The choice is yours.

❈ Corrupt politics begin with you. Let go of manipulations, agendas, and other expressions of wanting control. Can you control your own mind? Try that.

❈ The chaos of the world is nothing compared to the chaos of the mind. It is merely an external projection of the mind. A quiet mind brings peace with it wherever it goes. The appearance of the world can go from tragedy to comedy in the presence of inner peace.

NUTRIENTS FOR INNER PEACE

GABA and **L-theanine** have been combined to make a great supplement called **Zen Mind.** It gives you a relaxed state of body and mind without drowsiness.

Magnesium by itself and in its elemental form relaxes muscles, regulates sleep, and energizes the waking state. It also seems to be effective in relieving headaches and migraines. I recommend the Natural Calm brand (www.naturalcalm.net).

YOGA POSTURES THAT CALM

Taoist yoga is a Chinese form of hatha yoga. The Taoists use yoga to stretch not only the muscles, but the connective tissue, altering the body in a more lasting way. Yoga becomes a means to open the body's energy meridians, but also to allow the body to sit in meditation for long periods without aches and pains. This kind of yoga will be very usable and beneficial for all those people who are practicing the modern office Tao of sitting in a chair behind a desk all day. To get the full benefit of this kind of yoga it's necessary to hold the pose for upwards of three full minutes. I recommend three to five. This is a great time to watch the thoughts and resistances of the ego-mind. Set a timer for the amount of time you're going to stay in the posture. Whatever happens, whatever you feel in the body, whatever the ego-mind starts saying, allow it to happen and to pass through you like a wave, but stay in the posture until the timer goes off. This can be a very powerful practice.

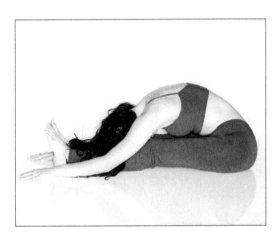

TAOIST SITTING FORWARD BEND

Sitting with both legs straight out in front of you, reach back and pull the flesh of your butt back away from your "sit" bones. Lean forward over your legs. If you can grab your feet, great; if not, it doesn't matter. Relax your neck, shoulders, back, and mind. Let your back round in this variation. The legs are straight, but you don't have to extend your heels as in some other variations.

The benefits of this posture come from holding it for an extended period of time, not aesthetic or alignment details. Letting your back round, as opposed to some variations where it's straight, helps decompress the spine and open your back muscles. Breathe slowly and deeply and hold this pose 3 to 5 minutes. At the end of this time, slowly roll up and lie flat on your back, breathing deeply for 1 minute.

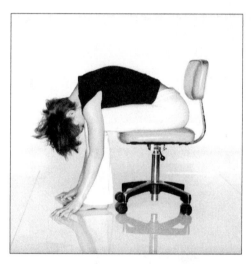

TAOIST SITTING FORWARD BEND—AT DESK VARIATION

Sitting in your chair, keep your knees bent and fold your upper body over your legs. Let your back round and breathe deeply and easily. Stay here for 3 to 5 minutes.

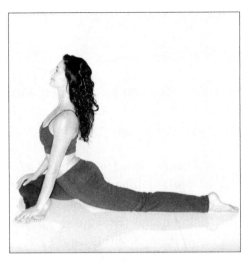

TAOIST PIGEON

1. From a cross-legged sitting position, keep your right leg bent in front of you and put your left leg straight back behind you. Pull your right foot up as close to the front of your body as you can.

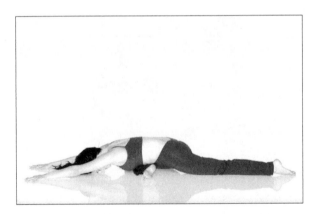

2. Bring your upper body down over your front leg. The knee of your front leg should be out to the side. You should feel a stretch in your outer thigh, back of the butt, and femur joint (hip joint) of the right leg. Relax your arms, resting on your elbows if you need to. Stay here 3 to 5 minutes, then change sides.

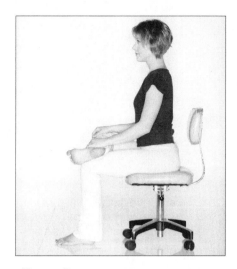

TAOIST PIGEON—AT DESK VARIATION

1. Sitting in your chair, place your right ankle on top of your left knee, opening your right knee and hip.

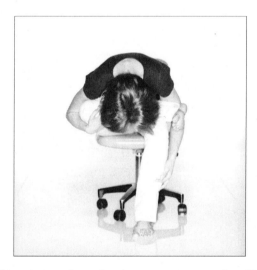

2. Lean forward over your legs, letting your arms relax. You should feel a stretch in your outer thigh, back of the butt, and hip joint. Stay there 3 minutes, then switch sides.

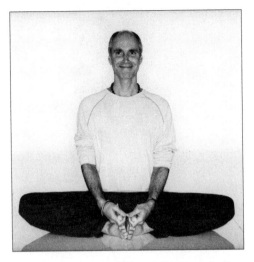

BADDHAKONASANA—TAOIST COBBLER'S POSE

1. Bring the soles of your feet together, pulling them in close to your groin.

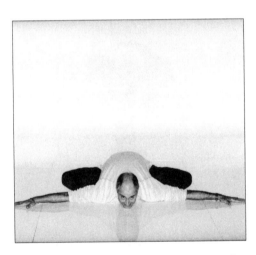

2. Lean all the way forward, stretching your arms to the sides. Push your knees down toward the floor. Stay there 3 to 5 minutes and breathe.

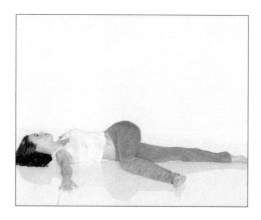

T<small>WIST</small>

It's good to do a gentle, prone twist for 2 or 3 minutes after these Taoist long holds. Then lie on your back for 5 minutes or so and let all of your energies balance out. You should feel very relaxed and open after these poses.

PLAYLIST SUGGESTIONS

1. "Grace" · U2
2. "Virtual Insanity" · Jamiroquai
3. "Revolution" · Kirk Franklin
4. "Come Together" · The Beatles
5. "Everybody Wants to Rule the World" · Tears for Fears
6. "Let Yourself Be" · Donovan
7. "Mysterious Ways" · U2
8. "Top of the World" · Brandy

One day, some people came to the master and asked: "How can you be so happy in a world of such impermanence, where you cannot protect your loved ones from harm, illness, and death?" The master held up a glass and said: "Someone gave me this glass, and I really like this glass. It holds my water admirably and it glistens in the sunlight. One day the wind may blow it off the shelf, or my elbow may knock it from the table. I know this glass is already broken, so I enjoy it incredibly."

—Achaan Chah Subato, Theravadan meditation master

✲ REASON 6 ✲

YOU WERE NEVER BORN AND YOU WILL NEVER DIE

Life is beautiful. There's treasure in every moment—treasure you may overlook unless you are aware of the impermanence of everything. Time, the physical world, and even relationships—which we have been taught to believe are the fabric of existence—are fleeting. This is the nature of phenomena: All that begins will one day end. Achaan's fragile glass is already shattered, but that doesn't lessen his fun with it. That it will one day perish makes it that much more precious while it does still exist. By living with an awareness of the transient nature of this existence, our lives become that much more exquisite and beautiful. Trying to force temporary experiences to last forever causes suffering. When a relationship ends, it ends. Why resist it? When a physical possession is gone, that's no tragedy. Didn't you have your fun with it? Then let it go. When a loved one dies, they're gone. So let them go. Didn't you love them fully while they were here? Didn't you share joy and laughter with them? When something ends, let it. It's the nature of this world.

In the words of the Buddha, "All buildings end in ruin, all meetings end in separation." *Everything changes all the time*. All of Zen points to that, all of Buddhism points to that, and all of yoga points to that. This is the simple truth. What you do with it is another matter entirely.

⤞ GET REAL ⤝

Death is a very natural consequence of birth. We come into this world in a mysterious way, and we leave it in a similarly mysterious manner. What is this fear we wrap around death like a cloak, trying to camouflage the inevitable?

At this moment in our culture, the mainstay of daily life is complete distraction. And the main distraction of the average person is the popular media. And the purpose of the popular media? It's big business to present trivialities with bloated importance. It feeds our desire to ignore what's truly important. Magazines for women are full of summer hairstyles and quizzes discerning how to tell if your boyfriend's cheating on you. For the men, it all seems to come down to a couple of essential truths: flat abs and how to have sex forever. It's almost laughable, it's so shallow. Almost. And yet we seem to live and breathe distractions, and think about them constantly. How do I make more money? How do I become a movie star so that I'm rich and famous and everybody loves me? How do I get a big house and authority so I can tell people what to do? What is that logic? (Hint: Egoic delusion.)

Everybody knows they're not really going to live forever, but you can push it out of your attention. You can push it away until it's so far that you almost forget that one day, it will all end: the story of your life, the body you've been keeping alive, your ambitions, your relationships. You almost forget that one day you'll die. That forgetting is called "going numb." Death terrifies you, you don't want to deal with it, so what do you do? Distract yourself silly. The trouble with distractions is that they not only distract you from the seemingly negative (death), they also distract you from the beautiful and miraculous (life).

If you venture out anywhere in the public today—a market, an office, wherever—there's always weird, whiny music playing, droning away independent feelings. There are stacks of superficial magazines laying around in every possible waiting area, readily available for the uneasy mind. The first thing many people do when they get home from work is turn on the TV. Even if they're not watching, they need the background noise if they're alone. These distractions serve to postpone our fears—distract us from potentially uncomfortable thoughts or feelings. To a certain extent, death has been squashed out of our culture. To the same extent, so has life.

If you get the chance to see some parts of India where they can't afford to gloss over mortality with magazines and Muzak, it will be obvious to you that death is real and unavoidable. People are dying all over the place; everyone's got warts, growths, and weird body shapes; but it's right there. It is what it is and no one's trying to ignore it. They just let it hang out all over the place, as they are. It's alive, not deadened by pretense. You see dead bodies, you see disease, you see people shitting in the streets. I'm not saying that vulgarity or poverty are good, but I am saying that if it's there, it's better to have it out where you can see it, deal with it, and acknowledge it rather than living in denial. In the United States, you don't see death, ever.

In the United States, old people are put away in homes where they often die lonely, closeted deaths that no one will have to watch. That way, we can all pretend that it will never happen to us. Is that sane? Old people can be such treasures when they have wisdom to share. But our culture doesn't encourage wisdom; it encourages consumption. Our particular culture is beginning to sweep the world, and as a result of this globalization, we're teaching the whole world to be superficial and better consumers. But is there joy? Truth? Awareness of the sanctity of life?

The yogis of India don't have much of a choice; they have to look death in the eye—it's everywhere. But even yogis who live in cultures where death is not so obvious make the effort to confront it. There are Zen monasteries in Japan where the monks do death meditation. The whole monastery goes to the local morgue and sits on the floor. Then they say, "Roll out the bodies." All of the bodies that died that day are brought out and put on display for the monks. The monks just sit there and look at the empty corpses. It's not sad or morbid, it's looking death in the eye. Someday it will happen to all of us. To know you will one day die is to know you are now alive.

Embracing death brings with it deep and lasting happiness based on the acceptance of life and its cycles. It's not, "Oh, I'm so happy I won the lottery, I've made it, ha ha ha ha ha ha." It's much more profound and lasting. When you look into your own eyes, you'll see a soul instead of just desire and drama. You become much freer and happier. To practice yoga is to face your fear. Go through your experience. Face it and let it go.

The reality of your experience in this body is that it will end, and realizing that in and of itself can expand your awareness. For example, imagine you're walking down the street, someone bumps into you, and you drop your expensive, delicious mocha java latte. Some of it spills on your Armani outfit and the rest of it is polishing the pavement. You stand there cursing your misfortune, damning the person who bumped you, mourning your ruined threads, and lamenting the fallen, spilled hot cup of java, possibly breaking into a sweat over the matter. As you contemplate the various other coffee shops in your vicinity, you suddenly witness a horrible car accident right in front of you. Your whole point of view shifts. You might feel humbled for getting upset over something so relatively unimportant. The awareness of mortality can shift our priorities, our focus, and our purpose in life. Yoga practice aims to prolong and sustain this kind of shift in awareness.

No matter how much positive thinking you do, no matter what your religion is, no matter if you do qi gong and yoga, dressed in magnets twice daily, sooner or later, the body's going to die. Maybe you'll be one of those miracle gurus who lives to be five hundred years old. But at the end of five hundred years? It will still seem like your life happened in a finger snap and your body will still die. In this universe, sooner or later, all things perish. In the words of Eckhart Tolle, "Even the sun will die."

What do you do with the knowledge of this mortality? Well, that's up to you. It can be motivation to search for what's real instead of wasting time on clothes, cosmetics, cars, sports, or who's doing who. You can focus the thrust of your attention on deeper matters.

There's no better way to distract from the fact that everything is temporary than the idea of happiness in the future. I live in Los Angeles, and everybody here's an actor (or an aspiring actor)—even the dentists, doctors, lawyers, rock stars, and many of the writers. They're all looking for that big break that will make them a movie star. "If only I could get that, or be that, I'd be happy, I'd make tons of money, I'd get the respect of the people I don't even respect myself, I'd get lots of approval and love, and then maybe I'd like myself." They are full of the promise of future happiness, which is sad because you can have happiness right now, right where you are. People waste away in Hollywood chasing that future projection of fulfillment. They can't see the fulfillment that's here and now—every moment of every day—because they're so distracted by the idea of someday. Why not be happy right now, right where you are?

Why not skip to the end? Skip all the crap and find out what you're distracting yourself from in the first place. Find out what you're avoiding. Go beyond the distractions of the world and find out what you're afraid of. Accept that you will someday die and cut to the essence of your life. Get to what's real. You're so much more vast than you can imagine when you allow yourself to be as you are.

There's a hidden promise in all distractions, implying that if you can attain success, power, wealth, or fame, you can live forever. But the true delusion is not that you can live forever, it's something deeper than that. The true illusion is that you are this body, this history, and this future, which was born and will someday die. You *will* live forever, but not the way you've been conditioned to believe.

Felice, a yoga student of mine, told me once of her experience with her grandmother's death. She had gone to see her grandmother, who she knew was ill and probably not going to live much longer. She had been apprehensive about being alone with her grandmother, afraid of what might happen when her body died. But as fate would have it, Felice was the only one in the room with her when she passed away. Had she known her grandmother was going to die at that moment, she told me she wasn't sure she would have volunteered to be with her. But once she experienced it, it became one of her most treasured moments. It was the most beautiful event she had ever witnessed. First, the room filled with powerful energy that she could feel—tingly like static. Then she and her grandmother both became very calm. As her grandmother exhaled her last breath, Felice said that she could see and feel the life leaving her grandmother's body. She said it felt similar to a birth, that the same way life miraculously appears, life miraculously disappears. It was in that moment she realized that the body is only a container for the life that occupies it for the period of a lifetime. After that last breath, her grandmother had gone somewhere else. That body became empty. Felice didn't cry for her grandmother. The only sadness Felice felt was her own personal desire to see her grandma again. She knew that her grandmother had made a journey and was safe and peaceful. She knew it because she was present when it happened.

This body and this particular story are going to end. You are not.

INNER YOGA

1. What do you try to hide or cover up about yourself? What do you think is totally unacceptable about yourself—something you wouldn't want anyone to know about? Make a list: warts, fears, things you've done in the past, and so on. Just in this moment, accept these things. Allow these elements to exist. Just for a moment, stop hiding.

2. Do you have any future-based desires—something that holds a promise of total fulfillment if you can attain it? How do you know that you won't be exactly the same person in the future that you are now? Imagine that you have attained your goal. How do you feel? What happens next?

3. See if you can feel fulfilled, loved, and happy right now, right where you are. (Hint: You can.)

⊰ THE BODY ⊱

The truth is that your body may live less than a hundred years. In the best-case scenario, the body may hold out upwards of 120 years if you're eating consciously, taking the right vitamins, and blessed with a favorable genetic inheritance. What is it that dies? Is it you? Or is it just the body?

The ego supplies the fears that when the body goes, you go. Do you think you're the body and that's all you are? You can try to sustain this belief if you really want to, but it's not that much fun as far as beliefs go. It carries with it tremendous trepidation, and all the associated distress that goes along with fear.

The yogis not only believe, but have experienced for thousands of years, that you're not just your body. In fact, in this lifetime you can separate your awareness from your body if you really want to. The yogis call it astral projection, and it's very common among yogis in India. There's actually a town in India that has so many yogis who practice astral projection that now they have to get a permit from the town to leave the body. That way, while the body is empty, waiting for the soul to return, no one will mistake it for being dead and bury it by mistake. To leave the body and go on a journey as the soul, with no physical limitations, free of the boundaries of time and physical space, is as relaxing as a luxurious ocean cruise. It's not a big deal, just a little romp around the universe. The body waits, empty, while you go exploring. It might seem miraculous, but it's as technical a skill as learning to drive a car. Most people are scared to death to leave the body, but the yogis look forward to it. According to Paramahansa Yogananda, "It's dissimilar and fascinating."

I met several yogis in India who astral project on a regular basis. There was one in particular who had an American medical doctor document that his body was technically dead for a little more than eleven hours. Astral projection is just a skill, with the understanding that you are not just your body as the essential, practical foundation. But leaving the body is not the ultimate goal. Eventually, that happens naturally anyway, when the body dies.

Why call it *your* body? How can it belong to you if it *is* you? The answer is in the question: It isn't you. The real question is: Who is it that your body belongs to? Who's aware of having a body? The body is just like a car: It's a vehicle you're in for a moment, taking you where you need to go. When the body drops, you'll continue and eventually get another one, if necessary.

Accepting the temporary role of the body can be an incalculable relief. Rather than denying and distracting yourself from the finite life of the body, and then flipping out when what you deny—illness, aging, death—comes to pass, you start to see all experience from a more informed vantage point. Your whole experience shifts when you understand that this existence, as it is, in this body, in this story, is short. Considering the age of the universe itself, the body is but a short breath, a wink of the eye, in the big picture. The death of the body is an obvious result of the life of the body, and you can flow with it. This is not to say that you ought to deny and devalue the importance of this life. Quite the opposite: Moments are fleeting, and we're like snowflakes or grains of sand—both absolutely inconsequential and utterly sacred. As with all yogic truths, both ends of the spectrum of duality are true simultaneously.

Once you realize the body's not going to last forever, there's a shift. The brevity of the life of the body can either send you into a downward spiral of complacency and laconic apathy (what's the point of living if everything's temporary?) or it can wake you up to the beauty, the perfection, the opportunity, the aliveness, of every moment. This second option affords you a slightly more enjoyable time.

You only have so long in the body, so establish your approach to it now. Yogis would say that you may as well take care of it and have fun with it. If you were going to be stuck in a car for the next eighty years, with little or no chance of getting out, you'd probably want to find out how to take the best care of the car, keep it clean, and find out how it works. The yogic tradition leans in this direction in terms of dealing with the body (and dealing with cars). There are those who realize that one day the body will die and they take a completely different, nonyogic approach. With a doctor's diagnosis of imminent death, some people, believing they have only two months to live, will go out and drink, take every drug, and have as much sex as they can. You can do that if you want to. Other people will go to a monastery to meditate. You can do that, too. Other people will just go on with their lives as if nothing has changed. That's an option. Some people will tell everyone, "I'm going to die, I'm going to die," and try to evoke as much sympathy as they possibly can. You can go this route, too. The reaction to the death of the body varies. But one thing remains the same: When you realize that the life of the body is going to end, whether it's in two months or fifty years, you become empowered with choice. Deciding how you will spend your remaining days can take your experience from an unconscious realm of denial and distraction to a point of relative freedom, freedom from thinking you are in control and freedom from believing you are this body.

When you realize that the body is going to die, you become empowered with a great freedom—it's a significant step toward dealing with existence of the body in a yogic way. But if you're not the body and who you are continues even after you drop the body, what's the point of sticking around? Why not drop the body now and be done with it? What's the point of caring for the body and extending its time if it's just going to give out on you one day anyway? If you're apathetic, spiritless, or have been hardened by junk food and carnival life, this might be your initial reaction. But hopefully you're not so far gone that you say, "I'm gonna die anyway, so I'm going to smoke eight packs a day, inhale cigars, and eat deep-fried hamburgers."

To the yogi, there is one advantage to staying in the body as long as possible. There's more time to dive deep inside one's Self in search of the truth and source of all existence. Your moments in your body are limited, but that makes them no less sacred. The body is the most limited, dense experience for the spirit, and as much as that can be problematic, it can be a precious opportunity. The human form and earthly existence are not without their challenges, but in all of the universe and all of its forms and formless existences, the body is the place you've got the best chance to become Self-realized. You're lucky to be stuck in one.

INNER YOGA

1. Consider the age of the universe. Now, consider the age of this planet. Now, consider the age of the room or location in which you are reading these words. Now, consider the age of your body.

2. What if you only had two years to live? What would you do with the rest of the time you have in your body? What if you had only two months? What would you do?

⊰ YOUR OWN PERSONAL TEMPLE ⊱

The desire to cling to the body and stay in the body generally comes from the fear that you'll die if you leave it. But every night when you sleep, you leave the body. If you don't think you leave the body, where do you go when you're dreaming? Try describing how the body feels when you're asleep. In your experience, there is no body and no mind. Sometimes you even relinquish your identity and dream that you're someone else. The world as you know it disappears. No matter how fascinating your life is and how much you love it, even if you've got a giant house, a gorgeous spouse, and a great job, when it comes time to sleep, you renounce everything. Your world dissolves and you give it up happily. Why? Because it's such a great relief to go to sleep and give up worldly attachments. The same is true when you drop the body or it dies. Just like you don't worry about going to sleep and waking up, don't worry about dying, don't worry about being born, and don't worry about living—it's all the same thing.

According to the yogis, the essence of living is this: Bodies, identities, and locations will come and go, but your Self is eternal. Your essential awareness has no beginning and no end. It is timeless. Your thought patterns and desires will remain intact within the Self until you choose to transcend them. A place like heaven doesn't happen in the future—it happens *now* or not at all. Find out who and what you are, and you can reside in everlasting bliss as long as you choose—in this body and out of it. If that's not incentive to stop putting off your quest for enlightenment and freedom, I don't know what is.

According to the yogis, a human being has four bodies: the physical body, the subtle body, the causal body, and the supercausal body. If you close your eyes and put your hands out in front of you, how do you know your hands are there? What do you feel? If you're able to sense a tingling—a vibration—what you're feeling is the subtle body. If you are quiet enough, you can sense that energy throughout your entire being. This is the eternal aspect of you—your life force.

The yogis explain that when you die, the only thing that dies is the physical body. The other energy bodies remain intact and go where they need to go. Your awareness, thought patterns, desires, and essence go with you. Then when it's time to take a new form, you get encased in a new body of skin and bones, and after squirming for a few months before you pop out of your mother, you promptly forget everything. You're back in the world again, and you again have the chance to dwell in the world of duality and possibly to wake up.

When you meditate, practice yoga postures, or engage in any activity with the intention of expanding your awareness, it's important to be conscious of your choices in regard to the body. It's not that you should obsess about your appearance. It's more about the vibration you sustain when it comes to the temple in which you dwell (the body). It's your temple, so however you see fit to care for the body and respect it will do. Some yogis sit naked on a garbage heap and throw stones and abuses at anyone who comes near them—that's one way. Or you can perfume it, pray in it, and live in it like it's a cathedral—that's another way.

Creating a sacred space, like a meditation room or corner, helps to maintain a high vibration in the body. If you go out into the chaos of the world—to work, run errands, visit relatives—it makes a huge difference to have a place that is just for being quiet and connecting with the divine. Like the body, a place holds energy. You can feel a shift in your awareness when you walk into an ancient cathedral or temple. Because people have come there seeking peace for so long, the physical location holds that vibration and the vibration takes you into a peaceful state. There are some temples in India where the energy is so strong you don't have to do anything except walk in and sit down. The temple meditates you. The etheric imprint left by thousands of years of peaceful intentions from all the souls before you is helpful. You can do this for yourself at home—create a sacred space. Create a sanctuary in your home and in your body.

Yogis—knowing the cycle of births is merely a play pointing toward the ultimate reality, enlightenment—desire to be free of delusion, know the truth of existence, and experience ultimate reality. While you're alive, use what seems to be time wisely. This is your big chance.

⇥ KUNDALINI RISING ⇤

Contrary to popular belief in the Western world, hatha yoga postures were not originally designed solely for keeping the body fit. In fact, their true purpose in the yoga sciences is to awaken the dormant spiritual energy, called Kundalini, in the body. According to scriptures, the postures themselves occurred spontaneously in meditating yogis once their Kundalini had awakened. While sitting in meditation, their bodies would just begin to move, taking them through these purifying positions and then eventually returning them to a physically still meditation. Other yogis, hoping for their own purification and Kundalini awakening, imitated these physical positions. That's where yoga postures originated. Yoga postures are only one tiny part of a whole system that includes pranayama (breathing exercises), bhandas (locks that move and hold energy), mental and moral constraints, and all sorts of austerities like meditating in rivers underwater for hours at a time, standing on one leg for years at a time, even drinking one's own urine (very austere).

The word *hatha* means "sun and moon," but it also means "forceful." It is an exacting kind of yoga, and it is for the earnest. What we do in the West are really just asanas, or postures, a small part of hatha yoga. The full body of hatha yoga is rarely practiced anymore, even in India, because it's so challenging. The hatha yoga system in its entirety has only one purpose, and that is to awaken dormant Kundalini.

Yogis attempt to awaken, or activate, this energy in order to achieve enlightenment and Self-realization. The word *Kundalini* means "she that is coiled," and the energy is said to be coiled 3½ times around the base of the spine. When this energy is awakened, either by long practices, meditations, or through the grace of an enlightened guru (the safest way), it starts to rise through the chakra system. Chakras are spinning vortexes of energy, and to thoroughly describe them to you, I'd need to write an entire book on the subject, so I'll try to sum up.

Kundalini energy and the chakra system are part of the subtle body, meaning that they're not flesh and blood. When a doctor is operating on you, she can't accidentally remove a chakra. Chakras are energetic and they remain with you even after you drop this body. As the Kundalini energy awakens, from the base of the spine, it's drawn upward, illuminating and energizing the respective chakras as it goes. Each chakra has a certain awareness associated with it; the base chakra is associated with survival, the second chakra is associated with sexuality and the senses, and the third chakra is associated with power. Most of the world is dominated by the energy of these three chakras (obviously). The fourth chakra, associated with unconditional, divine love, is near the heart, and the fifth chakra, in the throat, is related to truth and communication. The vision of the divine and clairvoyance is in the sixth chakra, located at the third eye. And when your awakened Kundalini energy reaches the seventh chakra at the crown, located roughly just above the top of the head, you recognize that there is in fact no difference between you and the source. When the crown chakra is finally stimulated by Kundalini energy, enlightenment happens. You become aware of what you truly are. In the words of Jesus, "I and my father are one," and in the words of the yogis, "*So ham, ham sa*," or "That is I and I am that."

While Kundalini is sleeping, its energy is the life force that animates the body and takes care of body functions—breathing, digestion, and so on. Once awakened, it still takes care of the basics (in fact, it takes better care), but it also revolutionizes your experience of life and begins the most profound leg of your spiritual journey. It makes what you thought was your spiritual journey, before your Kundalini was awake, seem like a trip to a grocery store parking lot. What was mental, a mere conceptual understanding of spirituality, becomes experiential.

I don't recommend some forms of so-called Kundalini yoga as they're practiced in this country. There's only one thing worse than never waking up your Kundalini, and that's wasting your time pretending to wake it up, or doing dangerous and questionable exercises that may in fact leave your subtle energies unbalanced or worse. Be careful: There are a lot of teachers out there who talk a good game, but have little personal experience. Hold out for the real teachers. How do you know a real teacher? Here's a checklist: Is this person genuinely happy? How often does laughter happen? Does the teacher make you feel at ease, accepted as you are, or do you feel not good enough? Do you feel a loving, blissful energy in the presence of this person? Is experience and joy underneath their teachings, or just an intellectual presentation? Do you feel peace in their presence?

Almost all scriptures, yogis, and disciplines recommend finding a guru to awaken the Kundalini energy, primarily because this energy is so powerful. Yogis have been known to practice austerities for an entire lifetime and still never awaken their Kundalini. They sit in caves and do mantra repetition for eighteen hours a day for forty or fifty years, fast for weeks and months, hold their hands up in the air for years without rest, all to awaken Kundalini. This stuff rarely works, but they do it anyway, hoping for a break. Without a powerful teacher, these austere tapasyas, or hardships, can be fruitless. Hardships by themselves just don't seem to do the trick. Some yogis have managed to awaken Kundalini by imposing this kind of suffering on themselves, but were typically unable to handle the power and went mad before the energy could do them any good. If Kundalini is awakened before you're ready to handle that kind of power and energy, it's like giving a race car to someone who can't see. Maybe they'll be able to figure it out, but probably they'll crash and burn. Having a guru is like having your vision *and* having Mario Andretti in the passenger seat telling you when to brake and turn. You probably wouldn't walk into New York City for the first time without a map, would you? When you've got a guru, it's like having a nice map and a personal guide to help you through what's new to you and what's old hat to them. It's all much easier and much less of a hardship with the grace of a master. If you can find one, it's a serious blessing to have insight and wisdom looking after you as you expand your awareness and come into your power.

This is the place and this is the life to do spiritual work. Yes, it's chaotic and there are distractions everywhere you look, but that duality is fuel for truth seeking. It's only in a physical body that Kundalini can wake up—and you've got one. The spiritual work that you do in this lifetime stays with you, even when you drop the body. When you die, your chakra system and your spiritual state go with you. It's a little slice of permanence, and yet it's so easy to ignore if you're focusing on what appears to be permanent in your daily life. It seems like a waste to spend your whole life focusing on temporary relationships and possessions and ignore your spiritual life, and yet that's exactly what most people do.

INNER YOGA

After you've read this, close your eyes and direct your attention toward the base of the spine. Keep your attention there and notice how you feel. Stay alert and be in a listening mode, paying attention to very subtle sensations. Next, move your attention upward to your inner belly, just beneath the navel. Notice how that feels. Next, move your attention to your solar plexus, and again, notice how the energy feels there. Next, move your attention to your heart. How does that feel? Next, move your attention to your throat. Notice what you feel there. Then move your attention to the area between your eyes, the third eye, and notice what you feel there. Finally, move your attention to the area just over your head, your crown chakra. Notice what that feels like. Take your time. This is a simple chakra meditation.

THINGS CHANGE

The only true security in the world is in the knowledge that everything changes. Every thing has a form and every form has a time span. And sooner or later (usually sooner), it perishes.

You can't cling to anything, because no matter how hard you try to hang on, life will pull it away from you eventually. It sounds sad, but in truth, it's beautiful. Life itself is changeless, but life expresses itself as change through change. Don't believe me? Ask any physicist. Without change, the universe collapses. You can't have a constant, stable, unchanging universe. That would be a nonexistent universe, an ununiverse.

The unchanging is what most people think they are running toward in life. It can also be described as security or answers. Psychologically, our human urge is toward safety. But safety from what—death? No matter how safe you are, death is going to happen at some point. So is safety really something to design your life around? Security in a secure world is an illusion, and this is where what is desired and what is delivered go their separate ways. And that's where suffering comes in.

The average response when you tell someone, "All meetings end in separation," is, "That's not right. It doesn't fit into the fairy tale that I grew up with. It's so negative." But the truth is that it's not negative at all. It's just an observation based on reality. It's common to believe that personal relationships will provide immortality—romance never dies! This puts heavy pressure on the average relationship. It doesn't matter what fits into a fairy tale because fairy tales are fantasies. And the fantasy is that you live together forever and ever, happier and happier, and finally the happiest. But expecting a fantasy to be real is like climbing the highest mountain and expecting to fly when you reach the peak. You have to climb back down. Happy endings are extremely unreliable. Happy nows are reliable.

Couples, for example, are nature's way of continuing a species. Even the most perfect, beautiful, romantic love affair or marriage is temporary. The fact is, sooner or later you separate. "Till death do us part." But you *do* part. In the old days, one person died before the other in the long-case scenario. Now, in our culture, it's more common to just separate, go to court, divorce, and then typically try to forget about each other as quickly and completely as possible. This is not to say that you shouldn't fall in love, get married, and follow your heart with lovestruck abandon. When you realize that at some point there will be an ending, you might see how precious each moment is and embrace your love with that much more passion. Take nothing for granted. Enjoy it while you can because it will end.

It may seem that you can control the universe and make something last forever: a relationship, a job, a physical version of yourself, or a social status. But you can't. No matter how passionately you believe you've found everlasting security in some earthly phenomena, it's an illusion. If you're trying to hold on to elements of life that are changing or have changed, extreme resistance and suffering can dominate your experience. Trying to make what's temporary last only causes distress. Yes, change upsets the illusion of psychological security. You can either agonize over this and fight it fruitlessly, or you can choose to pierce through the illusion to the truth.

So what is eternal? The life that's eternal is not a thing. What is eternal is the source of all things. Things—the expressions of life—are absolutely volatile and temporal, just phenomena dancing for a moment and fleeting. But the source of those expressions is absolutely constant. It's the only unchanging element there is. Life itself is not an object; all objects and phenomena arise from life. The source is eternal, formless, and beyond all effective conceptualizations. And the source is life itself.

Intellectually understanding that all things must pass is only the tip of the iceberg, but a very important first step. Surprisingly, though it surrounds us, most people don't gain personal insight into the nature of change. They have to read about it (like you just did) or hear about it somewhere. "Everything changes" is a very popular breakup speech, although I wouldn't say the end of a relationship is the best time to enlighten someone. If you resist the understanding of change, or you never hear it and you just go along with the old ideas—"I can control this and make it last forever" or "I just need more possessions to be happy"—then you go on resisting change and keep on suffering. Everything does change and there's no reason to lament it. It's okay. People hear it all the time, see it all the time, and experience it all the time, but once you really get it—and I mean you *really* get it—it's just so obviously true. Even the most resistant mind can't say otherwise. The most casual observation of life is full of proof that everything is changing all the time. From this very simple understanding, there can be a profound opening and a shift in your experience of living each day.

The whole point of yogic awareness is to put an end to suffering. First, you become aware that it's possible to transcend misery. Then, you have to see if you're suffering and over what. Look at your life, notice how, where, and when you resist change, desiring things to be different than they are. Is your life essentially just one big exercise in resisting change? When you start to notice what you resist, from there you can have some understanding of how you can transcend it. Like the yogis say, you can't get out of prison unless you know you're in it, and the prison is the illusion that you can push the universe around. The illusion is that the universe or God cares about your ego's desires, and it doesn't at all. If you go up on the roof and say, "I don't believe in gravity," and you jump, gravity doesn't care what you believe, and off you go. In the same way, if you resist change, and you say, "Well, I should be this, and they should be that," you just suffer needlessly. Understanding this is paramount. It provides enough of an opening for you to say, "How do I go about undoing this mess?" And the how is basically very simple: You just start accepting change. And you start right now.

INNER YOGA

1. Is there anything in your life that you cling to for security? If so, what? What do you think would happen if you let go of clinging? Who would you be then?

2. Notice what has come and gone in your life. It can be helpful to look through old photo albums. How have you changed?

3. Knowing that everything that comes into being will also pass away, how do you feel in this moment? What if everything in your life disappeared—your friends, your job, your family, your house, your money, and so on? Who would you be then? What would be left of you? What is permanent? Who are you really?

⊰ ACCEPTANCE ⊱

Right or wrong,
Joy or sorrow,
These are of the mind only.
They are not yours.
You are everywhere,
Forever free.
—Ashtavakra Gita

Temporary despair might result from the realization that even the aspects of your life you love dearly will someday change. This feeling will pass quickly if you let it. Cars break, houses burn, people change, pets die, you'll lose your body eventually, and the only element that remains the same is your *awareness* of this change. Any effort you make to cling is pointless, like spitting in the wind. Despair can dissolve, resulting in an entire reorchestration of your energy, revealing abundant power and freedom, if you ride it to its natural conclusion.

When you start coming from acceptance rather than the standard, chronic state of resistant, nonacceptance, your experience of life can't be stopped from totally changing for the better.

Happiness is a function of acceptance. You won't be flipping out about every little thing when you're accepting the moment as it arrives. For example, when you get something you really, really want, you accept it fully with no resistance. And you're happy to have it, right? It's not the thing that makes you happy, it's the acceptance. Two people could receive the same blueberry snowcone, and one will hate it and be miserable about it because he *wanted* cherry. The other will love it and be happy, accepting it totally because he *wanted* blueberry. If you can accept anything and everything, you'll be blissfully happy all the time. When you get what you want, for a moment your resistance mechanism is disabled. For a moment, you're accepting what is. Then, once that's over, your resistance comes back and you're back to normal. If your resistance didn't come back, then what would happen? You'd be happy all the time.

A common misunderstanding of acceptance is that it's complacency. It is not complacency. Acceptance doesn't mean that when someone cuts in front of you in line at the grocery store, you just take it like a doormat. No, acceptance in that situation could mean accepting the line hopper's transgression, then accepting the words coming out of your mouth, "Hey, man, the line's back there," then accepting his apology and resuming your place in line. Then not giving it another thought as you wait to be checked out. Easy, no problem. There's no emotional reaction to express or suppress, just a calm witnessing of the situation at hand.

Or, say, for example, you're driving along and you get a flat tire. The standard reaction would go something like this: "Oh, shit, oh, no." Then you get out and look and you think, *Oh, no, I'm on the freeway and it's night. Oh, God, my cell phone's dead, and I have to walk to the phone. This is terrible, so terrible! Why did this happen to me?!!* That's a scary story, and stress city for a few hours. The alternative? You can simply look out the window and say, "Oh, flat tire, okay, gotta walk to the phone." Then you walk to the phone. You're having a nice little walk. Then you make the call, then you sit in the car, and you're relaxed and at ease. Then the road service people come and change the tire, and *wwwsssht*, you're gone. Sure you could be completely insane about it and make yourself nuts and cry and weep and kick the car, and that's what most people do—about everything. But what's the point? Tires are temporary, everything is temporary. That's how it goes with temporary things: They come and they go. Life goes on.

When you can accept what is, the mental noise that fights everything all the time and the endless, chronic conversation in the mind slows way down. And when that happens, you become truly sane. When you *choose* to think, your thoughts are clearer. You're no longer just a walking, talking mental noise machine.

INNER YOGA

1. Is there anything in your life that you're resisting? Consider this carefully. What would happen if you accepted it?

2. Is there anything in *this moment* that you're resisting physically, emotionally, or otherwise—sounds, sensations, smells, thoughts? What would happen if you stopped resisting? Try it now.

⊰ **RISE TO THE OCCASION** ⊱

At the end of your life, when you look back at your experience, if you haven't grown substantially, you've really sold yourself short. Life on earth in a body is an exceptionally rare opportunity for transformation.

Big changes in life experience can be major wake-up calls. Sometimes life just throws you a curve ball, and in that pitch is the opportunity to accept the moment and grow from it. Some rise to the occasion: some do not. For example, the great modern-day spiritual teacher, Eckhart Tolle, spiritually awakened from horrendous suffering. His personal torture became so overwhelming that his ego snapped. He couldn't stand his own reactive mind and he was thinking, *I just can't stand to live with myself any longer!* And then he began to wonder, *Who is this self that I can't live with?* He realized that he was the one aware of the torturous ego. He realized that he was not the ego. He popped into what you could call an altered state, but really it's the natural, enlightened state. He describes it this way, "Enlightenment . . . is simply your natural state of felt oneness with being." The yogis call it Sahaja Samadhi, the natural, open-eyed awareness of one's true nature.

Thanks to the temporary nature of duality, you can get there in a natural way, simply by accepting everything instead of resisting everything—without ever meditating or entering a spiritual life. If you can stay truly accepting as your world shifts and morphs, and if you can face it head-on and stay alert and awake, the acceptance of change can take you to a high spiritual realization on its own.

The impermanence of this world pushes just the right buttons, egging you on to grow. Something's going to give, and the more you cling, the more you will suffer. Perhaps what you perceive to be great will happen to you, but even those experiences will end. Everything cycles through so-called good and bad, good and bad, good and bad. Problems arise when you think it should all be good, and you react, complain, manipulate, and control when things are bad. Get over it! Of course there's going to be bad along with the good. This is the world! If you win the lottery, you're not likely to think about deep spiritual matters while money is dumped on your front porch. You're probably not wondering, *Who am I? Why am I here?* It's only when you get the news from the doctor that you've got two years to live because you have cancer that you suddenly start searching your soul for answers. Money's a lot easier to accept than cancer. But cancer's more likely to start you searching for the ultimate truth.

When you're out shopping for jewelry and clothes, you're probably not seeking to know your soul or realize your identity beyond the body. You're more likely to be seeking a blowout sale, if you're seeking at all. Generally, you're just distracting yourself. But if one of your children died or one of your parents died, it could be a loud alarm dragging you out of deep sleep. Not everyone sees changes like these as chances to wake up. Change that seems unacceptable and leads to pain can be a great motivator for soul-searching. It's a vehicle for depth and freedom, or it's a vehicle for more suffering. You must either accept the change or suffer endlessly. That's duality, and that's powerful.

Resisting what is only serves to attract more of what you resist into your experience. It's as if the universe is pushing you toward acceptance by delivering the unacceptable. On the other hand, as you begin living life from a place of acceptance rather than resistance, so-called bad things rarely happen. Somehow, the universe knows that you're on the right track, and it supports you, making life a pleasure.

Being in a body is the most dense, difficult, challenging, dualistic experience available. It offers the opportunity for the most horrible, difficult experience or for the most heavenly, blissful experience. The extent of a person's evolution is proportionate to their acceptance of the unacceptable.

INNER YOGA

1. If everything is here for your growth, what are the situations in your life teaching you right now?

2. What are your favorite distractions? Make a list. Are there particular issues that really set you off and give you the urge to shop, drink, watch TV, or the like? What are these issues? Make another list.

3. The next time one of your least favorite issues comes up, instead of immediately going for a distraction, try allowing the issue to be there. Just sit with it, watch it, allow yourself to feel whatever you need to feel, and then watch it all pass away. Breathe. Allow. You'll survive feeling the emotion. Let it be without running away from it mentally (or any other way).

⊰ **START** ⊱

Teachers open the door, but you must enter by yourself.
—Chinese proverb

How can you be alert enough to accept every little thing? Start meditating. Ask yourself the important questions: Why am I here? What am I doing? What am I? Don't blindly take other people's answers—examine yourself. Don't get brainwashed by anybody else's opinions (including mine) about the real you. Find your own answers. Change will point you and push you in the right direction. The ultimate answer is within you and has always been there, waiting for you to get wise enough to start looking for it.

Before you get into a cycle of suffering (if it's not too late), start searching now. There is no other time. Spiritual life is about transcending agony, not enduring more of it. You don't have to wait around for the world to kick you in the teeth to start searching. Start searching when things are good. Start when you still have vitality, vigor, bounce, and peppiness. Don't wait until you're old and trembling to wonder why you're here. You see a lot of older people in churches, willing to accept any answer because they're scared of dying. Take advantage of whatever youth you've got. When we're young, we tend to go for as much pleasure as we can get (in between sleeping and work). Have your fun, but even in the midst of all that, look into the ultimate mystery. Get to the bottom of it.

There's an easy way and a hard way. The easy way is to be conscious, alert, and accepting. The hard way involves resisting everything and being normal (distracting yourself until the last second). The choice seems to be yours.

INNER YOGA

Have you had any hardship in your life? (If not, you're lying to yourself.) What did it do to you? Did you bury yourself in suffering? Did it serve as a wake-up call for you? Or both?

PRACTICAL TIPS FOR MAKING THE MOST OF THE TEMPORARY

❈ The easy way . . . involves accepting what is, being open, asking questions, being alert, and being conscious.

❈ The hard way . . . involves resisting what is, complaining, thinking compulsively, becoming addicted to suffering, constantly indulging in distractions, and denial.

❋ You are . . . eternal, birthless, deathless, beautiful spirit. You are one with all that is.

❋ Your physical body . . . is a temple housing the real you, which is eternal.

❋ Skip to the end . . . and allow yourself to be as you are.

❋ Don't take . . . other people's answers (including mine!). Examine yourself. Experience yourself.

❋ According to the yogis . . . the world is the place you come to grow spiritually. Don't waste a golden opportunity.

❋ Everything . . . is temporary. Trying to force what's temporary to last is impossible and only causes more distress.

❋ Your life . . . as you know it will end someday, so you may as well enjoy it incredibly while you can.

SUPPLEMENTS TO ENHANCE AND EXTEND LIFE

CoQ10 is necessary for energy production in cells. As the body ages, it produces less of it, resulting in degenerative conditions. By taking a supplement, you can slow down the symptoms of aging, including the breaking down of the body. It's excellent for the heart, brain, and overall energy. The liquid versions are generally more effectively absorbed by the body than the powders.

Thymic protein A (ProBoost) is also a powerful immune stimulant and prevents many of the symptoms of aging.

Oregano oil is a powerful antioxidant, as well as being one of the few substances effective in moving heavy metals out of the body (from air pollution, water pollution, dentistry, and so on).

YOGA POSTURES FOR LONGEVITY

It's a great gift to be in the body, and the yogi wants to stay in it as long as possible. Until you reach enlightenment, you want to hang on to it and prevent it from becoming a distraction.

The following poses are inverted and sustainable for several minutes. By reversing the position of the body, you also reverse the flow of gravity and its effects on the body.

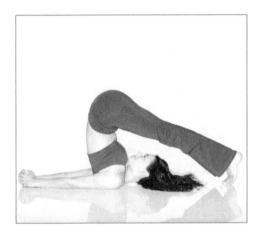

HALASANA (PLOUGH)

Lie flat on your back, and slowly raise your legs up and over your head, bending your knees if you have to. Ideally, try touching your toes to the floor behind you with your legs straight. If you can't touch the floor with your toes, just keep your legs straight anyway, not touching the floor. Support your back with your hands, or interlock your hands on the floor if you like. Don't force it; just go to a comfortable place and breathe. Hold it for 1 or 2 minutes. When you're ready, very slowly roll your spine down, bending your knees on the way. Squeeze your knees into your chest. Or, if you want to work your stomach and back more, keep your legs straight as you roll down.

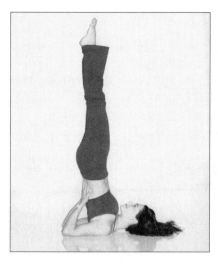

SARVANGASANA (SHOULDER STAND)

This pose transitions smoothly from the Plough. Once you're in the Plough and your hands are already supporting your back, simply lift your legs straight up in the air so that you're inverted. You want to equally distribute your weight between your elbows, shoulders, and head. It's not a neck stand, so don't balance all of the weight on your neck. (Also, you can fold a blanket and put it underneath your shoulders, elevating them slightly, with your head on the floor to make it easier on your neck.) Hold this pose anywhere from 2 to 5 minutes. When you're ready to come down, ease back into the Plough, or bend your knees around your ears. Then slowly roll down your spine.

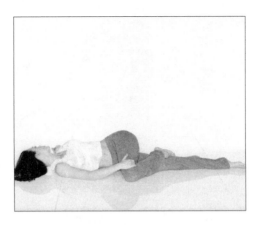

Twist

After the two previous postures, lie on your back for a minute, and then do a simple twist by pulling one knee to your chest and dropping it over the other leg, the toe near the kneecap.

PLAYLIST SUGGESTIONS

1. "Landslide" · Fleetwood Mac
2. "Wild Child" · Enya
3. "End of the Line" · Traveling Wilburys
4. "God Only Knows" · Beach Boys
5. "My Sweet Lord" · George Harrison
6. "Secret of Life" · James Taylor
7. "Everlasting Love" · Natalie Cole

I am no longer the wave of consciousness thinking itself separated from the sea of cosmic consciousness. I am the ocean of spirit that has become the wave of human life.

—Paramahansa Yogananda

REASON 7

TO THE YOGI, EVERYTHING IS BLISS

The enlightened yogis who have come out of India for thousands of years all arrived at the same blissful conclusion spontaneously. They swim in bliss, eat in bliss, live in bliss. They're blissful all of the time, whether laughing, crying, thinking, or not thinking. To the enlightened yogi, the world is ultimately just one big throbbing awareness of bliss.

Throughout this book, I've dealt with some common obstacles to experiencing the highest, most fulfilling version of yourself. Essentially, when you are no longer afraid of the world and when you are no longer desperately craving fulfillment from the world, there is truly nothing to worry about. And that's an extremely powerful position to find yourself in. Toward the ultimate yogic goal of enlightenment, this undoing of worry creates space for bliss and joy to gain momentum in your life, until eventually uninterrupted happiness is your predominant state.

This chapter will reveal the most essential adjustments that you can make toward not only removing worry from your life, but toward reaching the highest yogic experience: enlightenment. I must preface this chapter with a warning: In the past, there have been yoga teachers who prescribed steps toward achieving enlightenment. While it may have seemed like a good idea, it has proven time and time again to be a trap for the student. The primary pitfall is in believing you have to master step two before moving on to step three, or the thirty-second dimension before reaching the thirty-fourth dimension. You don't. Some serious yoga students have spent lifetimes trying to master step three, never reaching the ultimate goal, which is enlightenment. That's not what I'm going for in this chapter.

The truth is that sometimes you just need to hear the right set of words and you realize enlightenment. You can skip from step one to step eighty-two in yoga. It's not a linear practice. Do not mistake the subjects in this chapter for steps. They are merely tips, derived from my experience and the experience of many other yogis, pointing you in the direction of enlightenment. Having said all that, there is a certain progressive movement inherent in these pointers. One naturally leads to the next, taking you deeper and deeper, closer to your true self. One pointer may work for you, another may not, and that's fine. Remember, they are all pointing in the same direction, so don't get stuck on the pointers. Instead, direct your attention toward what they point to.

Every person on this planet is fully capable of attaining enlightenment. Even though it may require effort on your part, it can be easy. For enlightenment to happen, you just need these two intentions: You must be ready to give up pain, violence, and stress, and you must want freedom. The ultimate yoga is that simple.

⊰ **PRIORITIZE FREEDOM** ⊱

Man must ever be intent on discovering the mahayoga that will reveal his eternal union with the divine.
—Anandamayi MA, great yogini saint

⊰⊜⊱

Imagine you're making phone calls from your office and you catch on fire. Knowing there's a large fountain containing gallons and gallons of cool water just outside, you might head toward that fountain with urgency, right? As you jog toward the fountain, a pal asks you to join him for some lunch. Would you do that first, or would you take the plunge into the fountain to put out the fire that's about to turn you into a piece of toast? I think you'd put out the fire as soon as possible, then deal with your other interests. Life is a lot easier when you're not in constant pain. The yogis say that when your intention to be free is one-pointed and burning like this fire, nothing will prevent your pursuit of freedom. More important than anything else in the world is the intention to become liberated. When you have this, everything else falls into place perfectly.

⊰ **FREE YOURSELF FROM ENSLAVEMENT TO** ⊱ **COMPULSIVE THINKING**

You search for God in Heaven and Earth, but you don't know the one who is right before your eyes, because you don't know how to search into this very moment.
—Jesus

⊰⊜⊱

Freedom is the power to act without compulsion. And to a yogi, true freedom lies in the ability to use the mind or not use the mind. If you cannot choose to turn the mind off, you are a compulsive thinker. Ever lie in bed at night, exhausted, wishing you could drift off to sleep but absolutely unable to stop thinking? Thoughts just churn around in your head, unproductive and unstoppable? Why? These are your thoughts, so why can't you switch them off? This is compulsive thinking, and like any other compulsive activity—compulsive eating, compulsive gambling, compulsive drinking—it's not good for you in any way. It's self-destructive and it dilutes the potency of the mind. If you are a compulsive thinker, then at those times when thinking might be necessary and useful, the mind will perform haphazardly, without clarity. As you learn to turn the mind off when it's in the way, you'll discover that when you do use it, it's more efficient, sharper, and clear as a bell. There are some situations in which the mind will be useful to you. However, realizing the truth of the universe, your true, essential nature, and experiencing enlightenment requires the use of a facility you possess that is beyond the scope of the mind.

Liberation is possible here and now, but not through the mind. Your awareness of the world is confined by the mind, not enhanced by it. It's normal to believe that the only way to experience life is through the mind; however, this is not true. To truly, deeply experience life, you must rise to the occasion and elevate your level of awareness beyond the mind.

⚜ THE MIND IS JUST A SERVANT ⚜

I'm astounded by people who want to know the universe when it's hard enough to find your way around Chinatown.
—**Woody Allen**

⟶⟩⟨⟵

The yogis say the mind makes a good servant but a lousy master. When I say mind, I don't mean the brain. The brain is just a physical conduit. When I say mind, I mean the part of you that formulates thought, logic, memory, and projections of the future. In this sense, the mind is just one aspect of the brain. In *2001: A Space Odyssey*, Hal, the computer, attempts to take control of the ship and through logic do what's best for it and its human crew. From the computer's point of view, the best thing to do is kill the human crew and self-destruct. It is the same with the human mind. When the mind takes over, it rationalizes and justifies its inevitable self-destructive and egoic behavior. Most people are so possessed by the mind that they don't even notice. They think they *are* the mind.

How do you know if your computer has taken over your ship? There are a few tell-tale signs. If you are possessed by the mind, when you have an idea and that idea is rejected or attacked, you may feel as though *you've* been rejected or attacked. Thinking you are your rejected idea, you throw all of the weight of your emotional egoic defense behind protecting yourself. You're unable to pause and realize, "Oh, that's just an idea in my mind. That's not me." Just knowing where the mind ends and you begin is a substantial insight toward knowing who you really are.

To be aware of the mind, as opposed to enslaved by it, don't identify completely with your thoughts. Just start noticing what they are (primarily a bunch of noise). Remain alert and watch the mind's tendency to identify with what it comes up with. How do you think? How do you react? An attack on your way of thinking is just an attack on a thought, it's not an attack on you. If you can see it as such, and if you can say, "Okay, that's just a thought. These are just thoughts rolling around in my head, rising and falling in my awareness," you're one step closer to liberation.

You're not your thoughts, but when you believe that you are, at that point your awareness has become possessed by the mind. The servant has become the master. The mind can take over and push you around. And if you've got all sorts of buttons to be pushed, you'll be easy to push around. The mind creates thoughts, beliefs, and concepts, and spends the rest of your life defending them against change, opposition, and "others." Most people have been enslaved by the mind for so long, they don't even know there's any other way to be. You can go through life arguing, defending, offending, wanting, worrying, and eventually self-destructing. And many do just that.

But if the mind is your servant (its functional role in this existence), when you need it to operate, it simply does its duty. It will make its plans. It will say, "Okay, I have to wake up at eight, go to the airport at nine . . ." Day-to-day reality is not a problem. When the mind is not your servant, when it's running without your authorization, then it's being dysfunctional. So unless you need it for something, turn it off. Learning how to shut it off is the most important, empowering thing you can do. When you can get the mind quiet, then there's a real chance for a peaceful existence.

What's stopping you from quieting your mind right now? What's stopping you from having the experience of stillness as soon as you finish this sentence? Nothing except your mind and its momentum. Is it too simple for the mind to handle? What makes the mind think it's so smart? Yes, the mind can balance a checkbook, play chess, and apply for a credit card. But happiness? Peace? Bliss? This isn't the mind's territory, although it will try to make you believe that it is. The mind is limited, but your awareness—in which the mind, among other functions, exists—extends much, much deeper than the mind. The real question here is: *Who is aware of the mind?*

⚝ YOU DON'T KNOW EVERYTHING (YES, EVEN YOU) ⚝

To know is to know you know nothing.
—**Confucius**

There are truths of existence that the mind simply can't grasp, and this is where the wisdom of not knowing comes into the picture.

The yearning of the soul to see the truth, feel the truth, and know the truth can be overpowering. When a five-year-old hears a loud banging and moaning coming from under the bed, she might think it's a monster. If you tell her it's the pipes, you know that she won't just take your word for it. She'll want to see the pipes, touch the pipes, and experience the pipes for herself. So it is with the soul. The craving to know the source, to know God, is behind every yearning you'll ever know, and it's beyond the capabilities of the mind. A small paper cup can't hold the contents of an entire lake. Similarly, the mind is not able to perceive the magnificence of all that is. You—not the mind—can perceive it. If anything, the mind will get in your way. The mind will try to keep you separate, miserable, and unaware of the truth: that you are one with everything.

Yogis try to transcend the mind and go straight for the ultimate truth, which is perceived through pure, thoughtless awareness. The mind is always there for you when you need it, but to experience the unthinkable, you must rise above thought. As a being, your potential to see existence and the universe is limitless. But if the mind is dominating you, you won't be able to see past the end of your nose.

It's like you are a canvas, and this life is the painting on that canvas. Your mind has the view of the tiny tip of the paintbrush: It can perceive one little dot of the big picture. The picture is so much bigger than your mind can ever comprehend. How do you conceive of the infinite with the mind? It's impossible. Think of the infinite universe: billions and billions of stars, billions and billions of galaxies and universes and suns, infinitely spreading out in all directions, and then at the end (let's say there's an end to the universe), what's beyond the end? Nothingness? Then what's beyond that? Maybe there's just more universe? There's no way you can think about it. The mind just stops because it can't go there. To even try to express this idea with words requires contradictory language, and the universe is just a small part of reality.

History illustrates the obvious: Existence is unquestionably not going to be figured out by any mind. If it were going to be solved by the mind, the great minds of world history would have done it long ago. The best the mind can do is accept existence as a beautiful mystery. You can get closer to it through art, music, architecture, or sometimes poetry than you can through the intellect. Only a fool thinks he can think his way to any kind of lasting truth. The ultimate reality is not rationally accessible.

When you accept that you don't know, there's an opening in your awareness, and it becomes possible to turn your attention around and look within yourself. Looking inside of yourself doesn't mean looking inside your body, nor does it mean looking inside your mind. The ultimate truth is not in your memory somewhere, and it's not in a concept or belief that you can cling to for a brief moment of security and consolation. It's in what animates your mind, the senses, beats your heart, breathes you, digests your food, creates the trees, the sun, the moon, the birds, the waters—it's life itself.

⊰ BE CERTAIN THAT YOU DON'T KNOW EVERYTHING ⊱

Here it is—right now. Start thinking about it and you'll miss it.
—Hung Po

⟶⟡⟵

There's a difference between understanding that you don't know everything intellectually and actually practicing this recognition in your daily life. When you realize that you truly don't know, a surrender to the mystery of life happens automatically. Living in this surrendered way makes life much easier, letting you get out of your own way. Resistance to one seemingly negative event can put into motion a chain reaction of several other seemingly negative events, snowballing into tragedy and stress. Acceptance of one seemingly negative event, on the other hand, and looking for the God in it can turn it into something close to a miracle.

There's a famous story told by the yogis about an old farmer. One year, he has an abundant crop. Everyone in his village tells him, "How great! How lucky! You are a very fortunate man." The old farmer looks at them calmly and simply says, "Hard to say. Maybe." Then, just as the farmer's very strong young son begins to harvest their crops, he breaks a leg. The villagers say to the old farmer, "What a tragedy! How horrible! Now your crops will just sit and rot on the field. What a terrible turn of luck!" The old farmer looks at them calmly and replies, "Hard to say. Maybe." Then the whole country enters into a war, and all of the young men from the village are drafted to go off to battle, except for the old farmer's son because of his broken leg. The villagers say to him, "How fortunate! How lucky!" The farmer calmly gazes at them and replies, "Hard to say. Maybe." The mind would like to impose judgments and values on the events of a life. In the grand scope of the universe and all of its activities, you can't know everything. Things happen; it's the mind and its conditioning that presumes them to be good or bad.

The life that flows through you is so much wiser than your little mind, and when you let life happen without resistance, without unnecessary thought, it goes better than you could ever have planned. There's certainty in realizing that you don't know everything. There's a yogic saying: "Let whatever is best for my spiritual evolution come to pass." Through that certainty in the perfection of the mystery, there's an energetic acknowledgment that you are part of a force larger than yourself. When your intention is set on attaining higher states of consciousness and when you stop second-guessing the unfathomable perfection of life, often those events that previously might have ruined your day—breaking your leg, for example—end up preventing something worse, or, even better than that, turn out to be the most transformative, helpful experience of your entire life.

Essentially, there are two ways to go through life: (1) Resist everything that happens and comes into your awareness, attempt to manipulate the world to the point of exhaustion, and think obsessively about yourself and your life situation. This option is predictable, repetitive, and promises suffering. And even though it's a popular operating mode in our culture, you don't have to live this way because there is another option. (2) Surrender to the perfect mystery and accept each moment as perfect and essential for your evolution. It's that simple.

If your intention is set on truth seeking, your experience will certainly unfold in a perfect, magical way. In surrendering, you allow the infinite wisdom of the universe to work in ways you could never have dreamed of. You allow life to surprise you. You allow life to be your teacher. There's integrity in being certain that you don't know, and there's a space in your awareness for real wisdom to find its way in. Some yogis call it "thinking with the heart." A moment may not seem perfect and shiny, but every moment is perfect, even in its imperfections. Leonard Cohen said it so well: "There is a crack in everything, that's how the light gets in."

When you know you don't know, there's certainty and faith in a higher power that does know. This might be threatening to the mind. It might rebel: "Give up my hard-earned right as the one in control? Who will worry about everything? Who will manipulate the world?" The mind should be threatened because the realization of not knowing obliterates the soul's enslavement to thought and the limitations of your awareness.

You can embrace not knowing now and avoid a lot of heartache and drama, or you can suffer your way to the realization that you have no control, that the mind won't save you. But that could take decades, even lifetimes. If a fool persists long enough, perhaps he'll eventually come to a point where he realizes his folly, surrenders, and has a transcendental experience without the mind's interference. But that's really playing the odds. If you're wise, you'll embrace the mystery right off the top.

⊰ BEYOND LIMITATIONS: PERCEIVING ⊱ THROUGH PURE AWARENESS

Your true nature is beyond description. It cannot be known with the mind, yet it exists.
It is the source of everything.
—Nisargadatta Maharaj

⊰━◉━⊱

Once you realize and experience that you can't figure out the mysteries of life and its play of events, it will be easier to open yourself to a whole new way of experiencing what is. Pure awareness is a way of perceiving that does not involve the mind or thoughts. To exist as pure awareness is to exist simply as your essence. It is through this perception that you may eventually gain insight into what you truly are, what life is, and what the universe is all about.

First, the mind must be absolutely quiet. Then, you must listen to *what is* with all of your attention and life force. Of course, having read the last two sentences, the mind may think this confusing and possibly negate it. But when you try it, you'll understand. But don't drive a car or operate heavy machinery at the same time.

Your true Self can be perceived, and that's what yoga's about—directly perceiving and experiencing your Self as that conscious, eternal, blissful energy that people call source or God. That essence can only be perceived through pure awareness.

It is extremely difficult to express this point with words because words are of the mind, and the mind is limited, finite, and can never truly understand the infinite. When words try to express the truth of the universe and your true Self, it sounds like a contradiction: You are the body, and you're also not the body. You are your identity, but you're also not your identity at all. Each moment is very precious and sacred and also ultimately inconsequential. The source cannot be thought about; it can be perceived through pure awareness and it can be experienced. Awareness is the constant undercurrent.

Like a movie happens on a movie screen, experience, colored by the mind, happens on the screen of awareness. The screen is a constant when you see a movie, no matter which movie. Otherwise, how could you see it? Similarly, awareness is a constant: Experiences come and go, but awareness is the infinite space *in which* all phenomena appear and disappear. Awareness is eternal and vast, and it's there whether the mind is moving in it or not.

It's very simple: First, silence the mind. Then just be aware. Awareness will take you where you need to go. Again, I can only point to it with words because it's an experience that words can't really touch.

The yogis have a method of teaching called *Neti-neti*, which means "not this, not this." Because pure awareness is impossible to express with words, what can be expressed is what it's not. *It's not* looking at a tree blowing in the wind and thinking, *There is a weeping willow. I think it's beautiful. My mother has one in her backyard.* To perceive the tree through pure awareness is simply to experience it without labels—to listen to it with every bit of your being, to experience it beyond the confines of the mind. In a state of pure awareness, it's almost as if you forget yourself and become what you are aware of. If you are purely aware of the tree, you forget your body, you forget your memories and stories, and it's as if you and the tree are one (and in truth, you are).

Jesus described pure awareness perfectly as "the peace that passeth all understanding." By seeing through pure awareness, you're deeply peaceful and ecstatic, but the mind can't figure out why. You open the door to experiencing yourself and the world as they truly are—a wonder of unspeakable beauty.

Enlightenment is the constant awareness of awareness itself, which is constant bliss and constant peace. Thoughts and emotions may play on the surface of experience, but it's all united with the ground of being, always present as unperturbed awareness. Just as waves may have different sizes and shapes, they are still just ocean. Awareness is everything.

⊰ SAMADHI ⊱

Nothing was, nothing will be, and everything has reality and presence.
—**Herman Hesse, *Siddhartha***

⊷⊱◉⊰⊶

The ultimate goal of yoga is the transcendental experience called *samadhi*. There are different types of samadhi: The experience of a silent mind is samadhi, the experience of yourself as an aspect of God is samadhi, and the experience of yourself, everyone else, and everything in the world as one living bliss-throb is also samadhi. Samadhi can happen for a moment, an hour, or, if you're very lucky, the rest of your life.

While *samadhi* is the word yogis use to describe these expanded states of awareness, the states themselves are not solely a yogic aspiration or experience. Embedded in nearly every spiritual practice and religion is some form of transcendence or salvation. The symbols, names, and stories may differ, but the essence is the same. Christian mystics, Kabbalists, Native American spiritualists, Sufis, Muslims, Buddhists, and many other spiritual traditions have the same urge toward oneness with spirit. In a study conducted by Andrew Newberg, M.D., and Eugene d'Acquili, M.DI, Ph.D., evidence was found substantiating that the urge toward oneness is programmed into our very biology. In fact, the experience of what may be described as an altered state—oneness with all that is, divine abandon, communion with pure spirit—appears to be as much biological as anything else. By scanning the brains of spiritual practitioners as they prayed or meditated, these researchers were able to observe common, precise neurological patterns in subjects ranging from Tibetan meditators to Franciscan nuns. Furthermore, when the subject reached the height of his or her spiritual experience—described as a trance state, mystical mingling with God, satori, or absorption of the self into something larger—the scientists were able to observe unique, precise neurological functions in the brain thus far connected solely with these spiritual climaxes. Their study proved that connecting with a higher power is as normal a human brain function as seeing with the eyes or hearing with the ears. The yearning to know the divine is natural and innate. It is inherent in the human condition. This study has since been corroborated by studies by Paul Ekman at the University of California San Francisco Medical Center and by researchers at the University of Wisconsin.

You didn't just take form to eat, drink, mate, acquire possessions, get status, and die. You came here to find out who you truly are. Enlightenment is the purpose of human existence. If that rings true to you, it could be because your brain is biologically ready and waiting for you to make this connection.

God is not a distant form, but is all around, in every tree, brick, sunset, laundromat, road, and in fact, you. The state of samadhi is not this knowledge or understanding, it is this *experience* of oneness and connectedness. You can experience brief moments of transcendence without entering it as a constant state. The yogis have identified several different types of samadhi, each varying in intensity and length: nirvikalpa, sahaja, and sarvikalpa, just to name a few. But there are really only two essential samadhi experiences: Self-realization and enlightenment. Some yogis feel that these two experiences are indistinguishable, that having one is having both. Other yogis, however, feel there is a difference. So that you will have the benefit of both points of view, I will distinguish between the two experiences.

SELF-REALIZATION

No special effort is necessary to realize the Self. All efforts are for eliminating the present obscurations of truth.
—**Ramana Maharshi**

Again, I feel the need to reiterate that Self-realization is impossible to capture with words. It's just one of those things, like tasting a mango, that you have to experience for yourself. I can give you a rough idea, but it is my recommendation that you make the effort toward truth in order to have the experience of Self-realization for yourself.

Self-realization is the experience of what you really are. Self with a capital *S* is different than self with the lowercase *s*. I'm not talking about the self that's involved in phrases like "you're selfish" or "are you buying that shirt for yourself?" In yogic terms, realizing the Self is the experience of the highest, deepest, most profound, divine aspect of who you are. And once you realize the Self, you also realize that it's the only true version of who you are. All the rest is silly fodder for stress, and not real at all.

Through Self-realization, you realize that you're not only close, intermingling, and connected, but *one* with the divine. In the realization of the Self, one sees him or herself as divine, that personal history is in fact irrelevant, the future is a perfect mystery, and an eternal now is all there is. This depth of awareness feels like being bathed in bliss and soaked in heaven, until the bliss seeps in and becomes your very being. You are a vibrating, spacious, calm breath of God, so perfectly alive and in love with simply being.

The taste of divinity gained from Self-realization increases the hunger for divinity. Once you've had the profound experience of being one with God, everything else pales in comparison. There's nothing like it. The bliss is so powerful that sex, success, drugs, and possessions all lose their compulsive pull. Nothing can fill the void and appease the hunger like oneness with the infinite. Compared to Self-realization, the material world appears intensely mundane and shallow. But from this hunger for more God, one can graduate to the deeper experience of enlightenment.

ENLIGHTENMENT

If we are not hampered by our confused subjectivity,
this our worldly life is an act of Nirvana itself.
—**Mahayana Sutra**

Again, words are of the mind and enlightenment is an experience beyond the mind. Words won't reach it. They'll strain to encompass such a state, but they will always fail. Nevertheless, they can try.

With the experience of Self-realization, where you feel an almost personal oneness with the divine, the contrast of the experience of the physical world—and sometimes other people—often feels like a mundane letdown. In the enlightened state, however, everything comes alive as glistening, pulsing consciousness. One completely loses the sense of separateness. The distinction of the you and not you dissolves. Time dissolves and there is only infinity; you are one with everything and everyone in existence; you are omniscience, awareness aware of itself. It is the highest union, uninterrupted bliss. You realize that you are one with the absolute universal reality, and the word coming closest to describing the essence of that reality is *love*.

The yogis say there's no such thing as an enlightened person, because once enlightenment happens, it's as if the person disappears. Of course, you don't actually physically dissolve, but limitations and suffering fade away. Everything is alive, everything is beautiful. Even a chair becomes alive and glows with life force. You naturally love everything and everyone, because all you see is you. You no longer identify with the body and mind; instead the whole universe is your form. You recognize your identity as all that is eternal, infinite, and blissful. There truly is no spot where God is not. You acquire a kind of X-ray vision: Where under normal circumstances you might only perceive a cranky, bitter parking-enforcement officer, in an enlightened state you see past the facade and recognize the radiance of God playing there. In a normal state, you might get upset if someone yells at you, criticizes you, or is rude to you. In an enlightened state, you will be charmed by their game, as you would be charmed by a two-year-old playing hide-and-seek. Your heart is full of love for them, for you know who they really are.

In an enlightened state, when you drive down the road, it is you, in the car, which is also you, on the road, which is also you, which is also God. When you breathe, the walls breathe. A frog burps? It is the divine, and you and the frog, burping. You are aware that you are awareness itself, the endless space in which all else arises and falls. You have no beginning, no end, and there is only a constant state of limitless love. From the outside, life remains the same, but from the inside, it is radically blissful.

I must emphasize that it's not an intellectual understanding. It comes from the actual experience that everything is a play of vast intelligent consciousness. Once you're in that realization, you see that one consciousness everywhere, and it appears as blissful play (as opposed to the pain-and-pleasure world). It's all bliss.

This is not to say that because the world is perceived as nondualistic, you can't tell the difference between hot and cold. You don't become insensitive; duality still exists on the level of phenomena. But an enlightened being recognizes and actually experiences everything as consciousness playing in and as form. Even though all forms are different, and some forms are interpreted by the mind as good while some are interpreted by the mind as bad, nevertheless, all forms, all situations, everything that can be experienced by the senses or imagined, is ultimately a manifestation—an expression—of the eternal. When you see the world from a state of enlightenment, you see the scintillating, vibrating, glittering, alive conscious energy, no matter what the form. Your eyes work the same, but you may see the actual vibration of energy in objects before you see the object. When you see people, you may see their consciousness first, then their form.

Essentially, you don't lose anything but limitations. You only gain bliss and insight. What slips away is the separate sense of egoic loneliness. All the fear goes, and any idea or feeling that you're vulnerable or can be destroyed evaporates. The fear of death leaves you, because you know your essential nature is unending. In a way, in this state of samadhi, you've already died. Your ego has died, and there's now only consciousness, awareness (the real you) revealing itself to itself in every form.

LIFE GOES ON AS USUAL, BUT BETTER

Wherever my travels may lead, paradise is where I am.
—**Voltaire**

◦═◉═◦

I have had questions from students regarding what would become of them should enlightenment happen: "Will I remember how to drive a car?" "Will I remember to feed my cat?" "Will I still be able to hold down a job?" "Will I hold on to the essence of what makes me special?" "Will I have any personality?"

The answer to all of these questions is yes. Life doesn't end with enlightenment. On the contrary, with enlightenment, you realize that life is endless. And your personality doesn't disappear, just those aspects that are dysfunctionally self-destructive. You will remain the same, but it will be as if you have opened a window in a stuffy room. You'll have heightened awareness and much, much more fun. But of course, your essence, that part of you that makes you *you*, remains the same. From the highest point of view, you can drop down to any level you choose. You can travel around the universe enjoying omnipresence or you can go to a Mets game—it is total freedom, after all.

I've met several enlightened masters, and the energy that flows through them is the same but each has their own distinct flavor of enlightenment. One modern-day master that I've met is very calm, sweet, gentle, and impish. Sri Nisargadatta Maharaj, on the other hand, a late master from India, would tell you about inner peace as he waved his arms around shouting and looking like he might take a swing at you at any moment. Both beings had the same experience and the same enlightenment, but the vessel it flowed through was clearly different. In 1993, I spent time with H.W.L. Poonjaji in Lucknow, India, and he would sit with his students all day, every day, guiding them and talking with them . . . unless there was a big cricket game on television. He had loved cricket before enlightenment and he loved it after. He didn't miss a match.

So, don't be afraid of these profound realizations. The only losses are of limitations and suffering. Otherwise, your life will go on however you want it to. It simply loses its urgency because you will lose your fear. Realizing that you are an infinite being in a finite vessel (the body), you will no longer fear death. Being totally fulfilled from within, you will no longer agonize over worldly desires. With no struggle to survive, life gets really easy. Fearlessness is incredibly attractive, and people will start wanting to help you and not know why.

Lester Levinson, a well-known enlightened Westerner, was a businessman in New York City in the 1950s when one day he was sent home by his doctors to die of various diseases. He locked himself in his apartment and began spontaneously inquiring into the nature of his relationships, including his relationship to himself. After several months alone in his apartment, sincere and wanting the truth, he had a spontaneous, profound awakening. Contrary to the doctors' diagnosis, he didn't die. When he went back out into the city, police officers, not knowing why, would give up their parking spaces for him (and if you've ever been to New York City you know what a miracle that is). With no collateral or references, a bank loaned him a huge sum of money, which he used to buy a building that technically wasn't for sale. He resold that building for several million dollars, spent what he needed to buy himself a quiet place in the desert, and then gave the rest of the money away. The world just opens up to you in such a high state. Fearlessness is in no way a hindrance to worldly life. Wise and so blissful that he looked like he was floating when he walked, Lester Levinson retained the essence of his personality—his wry, New Yorker humor, his silliness, his appreciation for the work of Tony Bennett and other jazz greats—but there was no more suffering there. Only bliss and love remained.

THE SNEAKY EGO

With the "I" eliminated . . . this is Nirvana here and now.
—**The Buddha**

An enlightened awakening can be so powerful that it happens in an instant and then never goes away. However, it's more common to get glimpses of enlightenment, and then through relentless truth seeking, the glimpses become glances, which eventually become long gazes, and then possibly a long-lasting view.

When you get a glimpse of Self-realization or enlightenment, it's of the utmost importance to stay very alert. The mind may try to make sense of the experience—which is impossible—and that's when you're the most vulnerable to the egoic pull, trying to suck you back into enslavement to the mind. Once the mind tries to figure out what's happening, the true samadhi ends. The mind may tell you, "I've had this profound spiritual experience, now I'm somebody. Now I'm very far above all the peons who are still trying, poor dears." This is a fairly obvious example, but you'd be surprised at the lengths the ego can go with spiritual holier-than-thouness. Be very careful, because this is one of the last traps and possibly one of the most destructive ones, preventing any real and lasting experience of samadhi.

The ego will try to creep in through the back door, so remain alert. The truth is something you allow—by getting out of your own way—in every moment. If you place the world, or worldly things like money and possessions, before the truth, you can lose the truth. In northern India I met a man who called himself a guru. He had fancy robes, long, thick hair, lots of beads, a very large ashram, and lots of servants. It's very possible that he'd had a glimpse or two of the Self, but I can't be certain. I do know that this guy had more pictures of himself posted on every wall, in every flyer, and on every page of every pamphlet than an American politician running for office. He was notorious for cheating people out of money, charging exorbitant rates for ashram rooms, and then refusing to maintain them. He gave away beads to pretty American girls, but that was the limit to his generosity. He was the star of his own little world, and he advertised himself as an enlightened master.

Let this man's situation be a warning to you. Would someone who is enlightened feel such a material lack that they'd have to cheat others for more money to fill it? No, an enlightened being overflows with the certainty of abundance. Would an enlightened being feel a lack of approval and try to fill the void with self-promotion? No, an enlightened being overflows with approval and love, and sees that there are no others, only the one Being in many forms. Was this man demonstrating separateness or oneness? He looked very unhappy and he was worried about all of his schemes. This suffering has the potential to lead to an opening, a search for peace. But by claiming to be enlightened, there was no longer any space for truth to grow. With no humility, how could help ever find him? With such a fortress of ego, how would he ever find deep and lasting peace? He might think he's really figured it out—he's cleverly accruing lots of money and everyone thinks he's a star—but the only one he's really cheated is himself. He's getting in his own way.

The ego is by nature self-destructive, and the most tragic part of egoic behavior is the damage done to your own inner state—the worry, anger, greed, and loneliness. The toughest ego to break is one disguised as and justified by spirituality.

The ego can sneak back into your awareness, possess you, and drag you into suffering if you're not very alert. So stay alert!

YOU ARE THAT

Real meditation is spontaneous. It is pure welcoming, because there is no choosing of whatever appears in the field of consciousness.
—Francis Lucille

The practice of yoga postures is not something you can do twenty-four hours a day, but the practice of yoga is. It may start on your yoga mat in a yoga center, but you can extend it into the rest of your life.

The yogi goes consciously, knowingly, for bliss, and the world goes unconsciously for bliss, trying to get it through objects, relationships, possessions, status, and so on.

All those things only stimulate a bit of your happiness to flash forth for a moment, and then it goes away and you're back to the realm of pleasure/pain, pleasure/pain, pleasure/pain. It's always only temporary. The yogic route is more direct. The yogi goes inside, toward what doesn't change, is constantly blissful, and makes up the entire universe: consciousness, love, bliss, unbounded awareness.

The true yoga is something you can practice every waking moment. How? Remember that you don't know everything. There is a larger force at work in your life and everywhere. Use your mind when you need it and don't let your mind use you. Don't resist what is—allow it. Happiness comes from acceptance. And make freedom your first priority.

Neti-neti—not this, not this—once you see what you're not, you might start to intuit what you are. Ultimately, you're not your body, you're not your intellect, you're not your feelings, you're not your emotions, you're not your memory, you're not your social role, you're not your ethnic heritage, you're not your gender, you're not your height, you're not your age, you're not your weight. What's left? The truth is, you're conscious. You're aware of being.

What's left to say? "I am that I am." That's about as close as you can get with words. "I am the witness" or "I am eternal consciousness" or "I am" are also pretty close descriptions. However you say it, you're pointing to the same thing: that which is prior to all identifications, prior to all expressions, prior to all manifestations in form. In other words, who are you underneath all your roles and beliefs about yourself? You are awareness. You are deep, causeless peace. You are dynamic, ecstatic. You are limitless. And even if you are not aware of it yet, you are free.

Everything is a play of consciousness—the divine, God, the universe. As you live your life, keep one foot in the world as it appears, but keep the other foot in the awareness of your essential divine nature and the truth of being. This awareness will deepen and deepen, and soon enough, promotions and weddings and warts and stinky feet all look like God to you.

When you've reached samadhi, you won't float around aimlessly. In samadhi, you will hear your calling, you will know in your heart, in your soul, what it is you're called to do—if anything. This inner knowing is beyond karma and full of grace. It's only when you're enlightened that you can truly be a contributing member of society. When the ego subsides, your very existence makes a profound difference. It's the egoic mind that creates greed, and it's thinking that creates jealousy and all of these other negative states. But when you're beyond the mind, life is beautiful and pure.

Just imagine being totally in love. You're not threatened by anything and you're not worried about anything. It's that limitless elation that has you walking on clouds, noticing beauty everywhere you look. Walk through life in love, with no resistance and without fighting what is. You're not in love with some form, you're just in love itself. Love's within, not without, and that's fundamental. It's your essential nature: You are love. Once you find it inside, it will reflect back to you from every form that seems to be outside yourself, and it will spread all over your outer life in a most beautiful way.

You came here, into your body and life, to find out who you truly are, and what that is cannot be written in a book. You have to find that out for yourself.

⊰ DAILY PRACTICE ⊱

Hold up your hands before your eyes. You are looking at the hands of God.
—Rabbi Lawrence Kushner

⊹⊱◉⊰⊹

You can practice yoga every day, in every moment, and you can also set aside a little time every day to focus all of your attention on exploring the truth of your nature. Whether you take fifteen minutes a day or three hours, you will benefit the most by doing something every day. Fifteen minutes of regular, consistent practice is better than three hours one day and none the next. It's the regularity that really sets up the magic. Regardless of your mood, your situation, your company, or your location, practice every day, and the rewards will be immense. Your practice gains momentum, and the peace from daily meditation flows into the rest of your day and transforms your life. Set realistic goals for yourself in terms of the amount of time you can commit to this kind of focused practice.

Most people spend hours every day maintaining the body—showering it, feeding it, exercising it, dressing it, taking it to dentists and doctors, shaving it, waxing it, and who knows what else. But the body is temporary. It will perish one day. Your soul is the one bit of permanence that you have, and yet it's common to disregard it completely. Try to spend at least as much time on your spiritual well-being as you do on your car, your body, your cable service, and all of the other temporary—and in the eyes of this yogi—less important, transient issues. Make your spirit your number one priority, and trust me, everything else will work out perfectly. Throughout my life, I've gained far more happiness and peace from daily meditation than from relationships, career success, or anything else.

I recommend creating a sacred space where you live. Set aside a pillow, a corner, or an entire room, and reserve this space for the sole purpose of spiritual practice. In this space, you will build up an energetic resonance of peace and tranquility. It becomes a sanctuary with its own powerful vibration of quiet and serenity. This vibration will help you open your awareness to peace.

Each yogi has four very useful tools at his or her disposal: (1) pranayama (breathing), (2) yoga postures, (3) contemplation or inquiry into what is, and (4) meditation. If you use these tools daily, you will find their benefits to be worthwhile beyond belief.

BREATH

Pranayama is a calming, centering way to go into meditation. I'd recommend doing five to ten rounds of any one of these practices before sitting in silence.

Nadi Shodhana (alternate nostril breathing): Tuck your index and middle fingers of your right hand into the palm of your right hand. With your thumb on one side and your ring and pinky finger on the other side, pinch the right nostril (with your thumb). Inhale smoothly and slowly to a count of seven through the left nostril. Still pinching the right nostril shut, also squeeze the left nostril closed with your pinky and ring finger. Hold your breath for seven counts. Release the thumb, exhaling to the count of seven out through the right nostril. Reverse. So it's seven counts in, hold for seven, and seven counts out, back and forth.

This practice balances the brain hemispheres, and leads to a state of deep peace and euphoria.

Ujayi Pranayami: Inhale through the nostrils while contracting the glottis in the back of your throat. Make a sound like the ocean or Darth Vader of *Star Wars*. Ideally, the exhalation should be about twice as long as the inhalation. Listen to the sound the air makes as it passes through the flattened glottis. This can be combined with alternate nostril breathing. The emphasis should be on making the breath slow and smooth.

Kapala Bati (skull shining): This is a forceful exhale and passive inhale. The stomach pulls back toward the spine as you exhale and it relaxes as you inhale, like a bellows. This rhythmic breathing can begin slowly and move to a faster pace as you practice. It is sometimes called breath of fire. Do twenty-five to fifty breaths. Repeat three times.

CONTEMPLATIONS FOR MEDITATION

All of these contemplations and meditations ideally occur in a quiet place with no distractions. Unplug the phone and close your eyes. If you should be interrupted, let that be part of your practice. Watch your reaction—don't slip into angry reactivity in defense of your effort toward consciousness. Don't be a reactionary—it defeats the purpose. Stay very alert. I recommend sitting in a comfortable cross-legged position with your back straight and head up. You can lie down if you must, but it often leads to sleep, and a yogi wants to stay alert and aware, so sit up if you can.

For at least fifteen minutes a day, sit in silent awareness of all that is. God takes care of you all day, every day. What's fifteen minutes out of twenty-four hours? Don't have time? Make time. Do it twice a day if you can. Be completely open; drop all of your stuff. Just be silent, absolutely silent. Quiet the mind. Don't move. Being still allows your prana—life force—the opportunity to slow down and even out. When it gets even and slow, you have a chance to experience what you really are. If you're always running around, talking, chewing, and thinking, your life force will be turbulent and disturbed. The only thing you'll be aware of is the most superficial level of thoughts and emotions. So get still. Calm yourself.

The following contemplations are good for leading yourself into a quiet, silent state after the practice of postures or anytime. They work only if you do them, of course. It may be helpful to have someone read them to you slowly, or record them yourself and then play them back. Be gentle with yourself and see what happens.

Where there are humans, you'll find flies, and Buddhas.
—Issa

⟶⇥◉⇤⟵

Contemplation 1

Never believe a so-called spiritual person who has a stern face and a furrowed brow. If he or she tries to tell you what to do and how to be, run like hell. I have been in the presence of many powerful masters in India, so powerful that if you're in the same room with them, you feel every cell of your body on fire with presence. If you say, "I have such and such a problem, what should I do?" this master will just laugh and laugh. That's all they do all day is laugh. What do they know that you don't? Nothing.

Contemplation 2

As far as people who are trying to live a spiritual life instead of a worldly life, it is impossible. Everything is spiritual. There is nothing that exists that is not spiritual. Everything you see, everything you experience is God.

Contemplation 3

Listen to the sound of traffic. Or any sound. The yogis call sound Nada Brahma, which means sound is God. The sound of that traffic is God energy. The floor that is supporting you right now is just a seemingly denser form of that God energy. Everything is spiritual life.

You may experience the world this way, or you may not. It doesn't matter. Someday you will. So if everything is spiritual life, what are you? (Take a wild guess.)

Contemplation 4

Everything is an appearance. Everything is an illusion. What you see is not really what it is—it is just an appearance. All of these forms are just one conscious energy dancing. You think everything is separate, but it's not possible, it's just not true. You think you're separate from everything and that's not possible.

There is no independent you. This feeling of being an independent, separate entity is called ego. This egoic presumption of separation is the primal and basic dilemma that characterizes the human condition.

All authentic spiritual paths and techniques are aimed at the reduction and eventual elimination of this ultimately fictional state called the egoic condition. Practices such as meditation, chanting, mantra repetition, prayer, devotion, and hardship of one form or another are all designed to free you from the slavery of the egoic mind.

Contemplation 5

Yogis say there are two kinds of fear: instinctual and psychological. Instinctual fear is when you're about to be bitten by a dog or you look down the street and see a truck coming right at you. That kind of fear is a legitimate link to survival and not a problem.

Psychological fear, on the other hand, is a dysfunctional state caused by living in an imaginary future. It needs a future to sustain itself. You have no idea what the future holds—no one does. Therefore the solution is to continually bring your attention back to this moment. For example, in this moment you're sitting here, breathing, alive, and everything's fine.

So, in order to let go of suffering that psychological fear, you need to continually bring yourself back to this very moment. If you want to see the extent to which people are not present, turn on the news. The vast, vast majority of people are dwelling in psychological fear. It doesn't help anyone or anything to feel bad. It doesn't help others and it doesn't help you, unless you enjoy feeling bad, which, though they don't admit it, a great many people do.

Contemplation 6

Toward the goal of freedom, yogis have recognized two basic human strategies: The most well-known and commonly practiced strategy presumes that you're not where you're supposed to be and that there's something to achieve in the future. So after lifetimes of hard work and much struggle, you may finally achieve it.

The second strategy involves the recognition that there's nowhere to go and nothing to get. Everything is perfect exactly the way it is. You're exactly where you're supposed to be. If you wholeheartedly accept that possibility, a big relax can happen. And from this relaxation, an openness and receptivity to what is appears. From this openness, with no effort, you find yourself in the place you thought you had to work so hard to get to. Freedom: It was here all the time.

Many people choose the hard-work-and-struggle strategy. And if you're one of them, all I can say is, good luck.

Contemplation 7

The ego needs enemies for its survival. Whether it finds an external enemy or an internal one such as a thought or a feeling, it needs this enemy to strengthen the fictitious experience of separateness, or a separate sense of self.

In this moment, see if you can relinquish that pattern and just remain content as you are, wanting nothing, with no desire to control anything.

To the degree that you can do this, your awareness will expand and you'll become happier. If you hang on to your discontent, that's something you're doing. Your mother didn't do it to you, society didn't do it to you, church didn't do it to you. That attachment to the contracted state is due primarily to fear. Why not let it go?

Whatever takes the greatest courage allows the greatest growth. If you play it safe, you won't get much. What you give is what you get. Why not be happy in this moment?

Contemplation 8

The yogis have a word, *maya*, that they use a lot. It's normally translated to mean "illusion," but the literal translation is "to measure." This refers to the mind's tendency to divide up the mystery of all that is into fragments, pieces, and parts, which are then labeled and dismissed as known.

This is why maya is used to refer to illusion, because the all that is cannot be known by the mind. Whenever you label something, you are deadening its aliveness for you. It's a superimposition of mind onto the beauty and innocence of reality.

Contemplation 9

1. Three yogis are sitting in a cave. They've been sitting in there for ten years meditating. One day a donkey walks by, looks in, and keeps walking. Five years pass, then one yogi says, "Did you see that?" Another five long years go by and the second yogi says, "What?" Another five long years go by and the third yogi says, "If you guys don't shut up, I'm leaving."

2. What did the yogi say to the hot dog vendor? "Make me one with everything."

MEDITATION

The following may be helpful for leading yourself into meditation. Quieting the mind and silencing your thoughts is the true meditation. I can't do that for you, but these lead-ins may help you to do it for yourself.

-→‒◉‒←-

Meditation 1

Begin by noticing how you feel in this moment. Bring yourself into the realm of feeling, not thinking. Don't think about how you feel, don't interpret how you feel, don't make a story about how you feel. Just notice how you feel.

Start with the body—the actual sensation of life in the body. The breath is happening subtly; perhaps there's a mild electrical sensation running through the body, various tensions, pains, sensations, heat, cold, tingles. That's all the physical body.

Now, see if you can feel the energetic body. By that, I mean the sensation of being alive. Your eyes are closed and you're just open to this moment, wanting nothing else but to explore this moment for yourself. Don't think. Feel what's happening, keeping your attention on the subtle feeling of life playing in every pore and cell of your body. Feel your aliveness right now and hold this awareness for as long as you can (even a few moments are extremely valuable).

Meditation 2

Sit straight and comfortable, eyes closed. You can open your palms and turn them up or however you're comfortable is fine. Just for right now, completely open to the unknown that this moment is. That means let go of the arrogance of knowledge. You know certain things in the world, yes. But ultimately, you don't know what anything is, you don't know what you are, you don't know what this moment is, you don't know what God is. What you might have are some beliefs, but you don't really know. In other words, the world, this moment, you—it's all unknown. So, open to that rather than resisting the unknown. Don't try to find some answer or relief via belief. Just open to the actual unknown in this moment. Whatever *is* cannot be reduced to mental knowledge.

Just allow yourself to be open, neither looking for anything nor trying to find an answer. Just surrender to what is in this moment. Open. If there's sensation, emotion, thought, feeling, perception, imagination, just allow it all to happen. Don't try to stop anything—watch it all as if it's a movie. You're open and yet watching. Stay with it and notice how you feel.

Meditation 3

Become aware of thoughts. They rise up, probably having to do with you, centered around the me: I need this. I want this. I don't like this. They're not treating me well. I'm not getting what I want. They're all *me* thoughts. Even if other thoughts arise—just abstract thoughts—see if you can find from where the thoughts arise. Thoughts come out of somewhere and disappear back into somewhere. Can something come out of nothing? See if you can find out where the thoughts come from. Be so vigilant and so attentive that not a single thought can arise without your catching it.

Really look and just dare your mind to think. You may actually find the mind doesn't think. This is one way yogis still the mind. Where do thoughts come from? Watch, alert and attentive, just as a cat very patiently waits outside of a mouse hole for a mouse to poke its head out. Like that, you just sit and wait for a thought to arise, and as soon as it starts to arise, find out from where it arises.

If thoughts like *I'm bored, I can't do this, I want to do something else* arise, recognize them only as thoughts. There's no need to empower them, repress them, or overpower them. See thoughts come and see them go. And see if you can find out where they come from. If no thoughts arise, you've discovered a beautifully easy way to the peaceful no-mind state.

Meditation 4

Science now tells us what the yogis have been saying for five thousand years or longer, that essentially all matter is just energy dancing at different speeds. For example, if looked at under an electron microscope, the most dense structures in your body—bones—are 99 percent space and a tiny little bit of energy moving, dancing, throbbing. If your bones, the most solid part of you, are that way, so is the rest of you. In reality what seems to be this dense carbon unit—your body—is actually almost entirely empty space with a little energy moving. It may not be your perception, but that's the reality.

So, in this moment, can you feel your own spaciousness? Can you feel what it feels like to be space? Can you feel what it feels like to have no boundaries, no center, no structure? There's awareness. And in that awareness there may be sounds, sensations, perceptions of the outside world, and perceptions of the internal world, but all these perceptions are witnessed by awareness. They're all happening on the screen of awareness. Can you feel that this awareness is absolutely spacious? Extending infinitely in all directions—front, back, top, bottom—there's no place where it ends, there's no place where it begins, just infinite space in all directions. The body is completely insubstantial. As a form, it's just space—oceanic. Get the feeling that all that space is inside of you, because all that space is in your awareness. You're awareness, so it's all inside you.

Allowing yourself to feel this expansion, take a deep breath and feel space go into space, and as you exhale, space goes out to space—just the wind inside of a sky. Stay here for as long as you like. And see if you can feel the unbounded awareness that you are.

POSTURES FOR BLISS

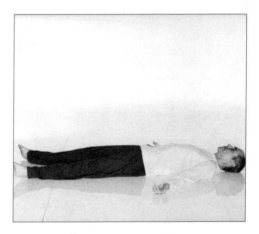

SHAVASANA (CORPSE POSE)

Lie comfortably on your back. Spread your legs hip distance or more apart and let your arms rest at your sides a comfortable distance from your body. Relax completely.

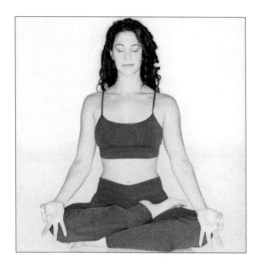

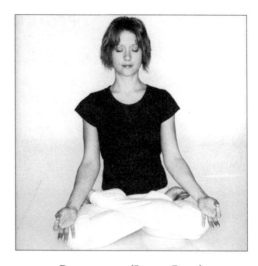

ARDHA PADMASANA (HALF LOTUS POSE)

PADMASANA (LOTUS POSE)

Sitting cross-legged, take your right
foot to the place on your left leg where
the thigh meets the hip.

Sitting cross-legged, take your right
foot to the place on the left leg where
the thigh meets the hip. Take your left
foot and place it at the point on the
right leg where the hip meets the
thigh. Keep your back straight but not
tense. This is a good posture for meditation because it allows a strong foundation for stillness. If it hurts your
knees at all, skip it and just sit in
Ardha Padmasana for meditation.

SPIRITUAL

Be As You Are: The Teachings of Sri Ramana Maharshi, David Godman, Arkana, 1991.

Deeper Thoughts, Jack Handey, Hyperion, 1993.

From Onions to Pearls: A Journal of Awakening and Deliverance, Satyam Nadeen, Hay House, 1999.

I Am That: Talks with Sri Nisargadatta, Maurice Frydman (translator), Aperture, 1997.

Miracle of Love, Ram Dass, Hanuman Foundation, 3rd edition, 1995.

Nothing Ever Happened (trilogy), David Godman, Avadhuta Foundation, 1998.

No Way: A Guide for the Spiritually Advanced, Ram Tzu, Advaita Press, 1990.

Play of Consciousness: A Spiritual Autobiography, Muktananda, Syda Foundation, 2000.

The Power of Now: A Guide to Spiritual Enlightenment, New World Library, 1999.

Silence of the Heart, Robert Adams, Acropolis Books, 1999.

Silence Speaks, Baba Hari Dass, Sri Rama Publishers, 1997.

The Bhagavad-Gita, Juan Mascaro (translator), Penguin USA, 2003.

The Gospel of Sri Ramakrishna, Ramakrishna–Vivekananda Center, 1985.

The Holographic Universe, Michael Talbot Perennial Press, 1992. (Page 59 to the end is my favorite part.)

The Kabir Book: Fourty-Four of the Ecstatic Poems of Kabir, Robert Bly (editor), Beacon Press, 1993.

Wake Up and Roar, H.W.L. Poonjaji, Gangaji Foundation, 1992.

HEALTH

Conscious Eating, Gabriel Cousens, M.D., North Atlantic Books, 2000.
Diet for a New America, John Robbins, HJ Kramer.
How Long Do You Choose to Live?, Peter Ragnar, www.RoaringLionPublishing.com.
Sugar Blues, William F. Dufty, Warner Books, 1993.
The Miracle of Fasting, Paul Bragg and Patricia Bragg, Health Science, 1988.
Your Body's Many Cries for Water, Fereydoon Batmangheidj, Global Health Solutions,
    1995.